T0373388

MINING THE HEARTLAND

Mining the Heartland

Nature, Place, and Populism on the Iron Range

Erik Kojola

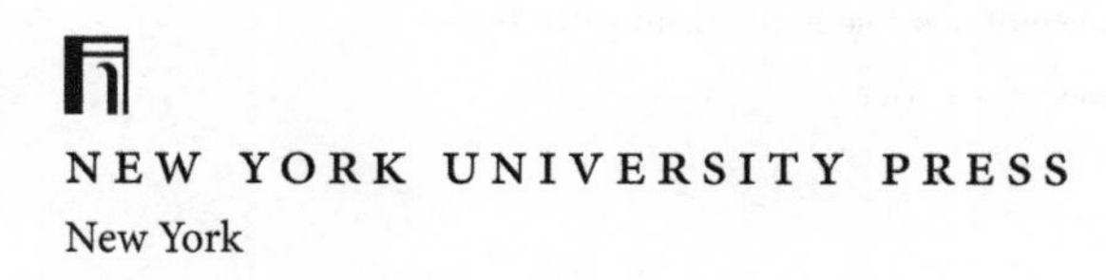

NEW YORK UNIVERSITY PRESS
New York

NEW YORK UNIVERSITY PRESS
New York
www.nyupress.org

Please contact the Library of Congress for Cataloging-in-Publication data.
ISBN: 9781479815197 (hardback)
ISBN: 9781479815210 (paperback)
ISBN: 9781479815241 (library ebook)
ISBN: 9781479815227 (consumer ebook)

New York University Press books are printed on acid-free paper, and their binding materials are chosen for strength and durability. We strive to use environmentally responsible suppliers and materials to the greatest extent possible in publishing our books.

Manufactured in the United States of America

10 9 8 7 6 5 4 3 2 1

Also available as an ebook

To my grandparents Rhoda and George, whose curiosity, compassion, and activism continue to inspire

CONTENTS

Introduction

A few hundred people gathered near a baseball diamond in a small neighborhood park in St. Paul, Minnesota's capital, to protest a mine proposed for the rural, northern part of their state. Staff of environmental organizations gave a series of speeches calling for the protection of "our water," a folk musician led a sing-along, and the group of mostly middle-aged and older white people set off on its midafternoon march in October 2015. Following directions from organizers to stay on the sidewalk and follow traffic rules, the group snaked its way along a four-lane road and over a highway overpass toward a semi-industrial area on the edge of downtown, arriving at a drab municipal building—the Minnesota Department of Natural Resources. Along the way, I chatted with a white man in his seventies, who talked about the project being risky and the need for more analysis of the economic impacts of new mining on tourism—a theme I overheard in many conversations about the threats that mining pollution poses to surrounding lakes. In the parking lot, an environmental leader gave another short speech about the need for rigorous government oversight and review of the potentially toxic mine. Organizers emphasized that the project would bring short-term benefits and long-term risks and could pollute people's drinking water and harm future generations. An agency representative, a white man in his fifties dressed in khakis and button-down shirt, emerged to briefly address the protestors, many of whom were carrying signs saying, "Protect Water, Stop PolyMet" and "Clean Water Supports Us." He acknowledged their concerns and accepted an oversized postcard of public comments about the proposed mine. He then walked back into the building, and demonstrators mulled around for a few minutes before drifting back to their cars.

Several months later, in the summer of 2016, another similar mining project was the subject of a public hearing. A mine was being proposed close to Ely, a small town of around three thousand people in the far north of the state with a quaint main street dotted with cafes, bars, a local grocery store, and canoe outfitters. The town sits on the edge of a mining region named the Iron Range after the massive iron-ore deposits, the Canadian border, and the vast Boundary Waters Canoe Area Wilderness (BWCAW). The BWCAW is a protected area with 1,175 interconnected glacial lakes and thousands of acres of boreal forest that attract people from around the state and country for canoe trips across the pristine blue waters and camping under the pitch-black skies—one of the few dark-sky sanctuaries in the world where planes are not even allowed to fly over. There, a rally both similar to and starkly different from the first took place at Whiteside Park, a small city park with a playground and picnic area. Local politicians, union leaders, and industry representatives spoke before several hundred people, who were adorned in "We Support Mining" and "Mining Supports Us" stickers and pins along with many union T-shirts. They extolled the proposed mine as a way to strengthen "our way of life" and as a state-of-the-art facility that would keep the environment clean while providing materials essential to modern life. Afterward, the crowd, large enough to effectively shut down the typically quiet residential streets, marched to the high school auditorium behind a banner carried by a Little League team sponsored by a mining company. People chatted and laughed with each other between chanting pro-mining slogans.

People streamed through the doors of the high school and settled into the large art deco auditorium—built in the 1920s during the boom years of iron mining—as it filled up with around eight hundred people. They were there to spend several hours on a summer evening listening to presentations and comments about the proposed Twin Metals copper-nickel mine at a public hearing organized by the US Bureau of Land Management (BLM) and US Forest Service (USFS). People gave impassioned two-minutes speeches (the time limit set by government agencies), many claiming that they were third- or fourth-generation Elyites and Iron Rangers, that their community was supported by mining, and that the new mining projects would breathe new life into the economy while keeping the environment clean. Yet there were also speakers—often from the city of Duluth, retirees who relocated to Ely, or owners of tourism-related businesses—who spoke in opposition to the proposed mine. Some of them were met with quiet jeers and murmurs from the

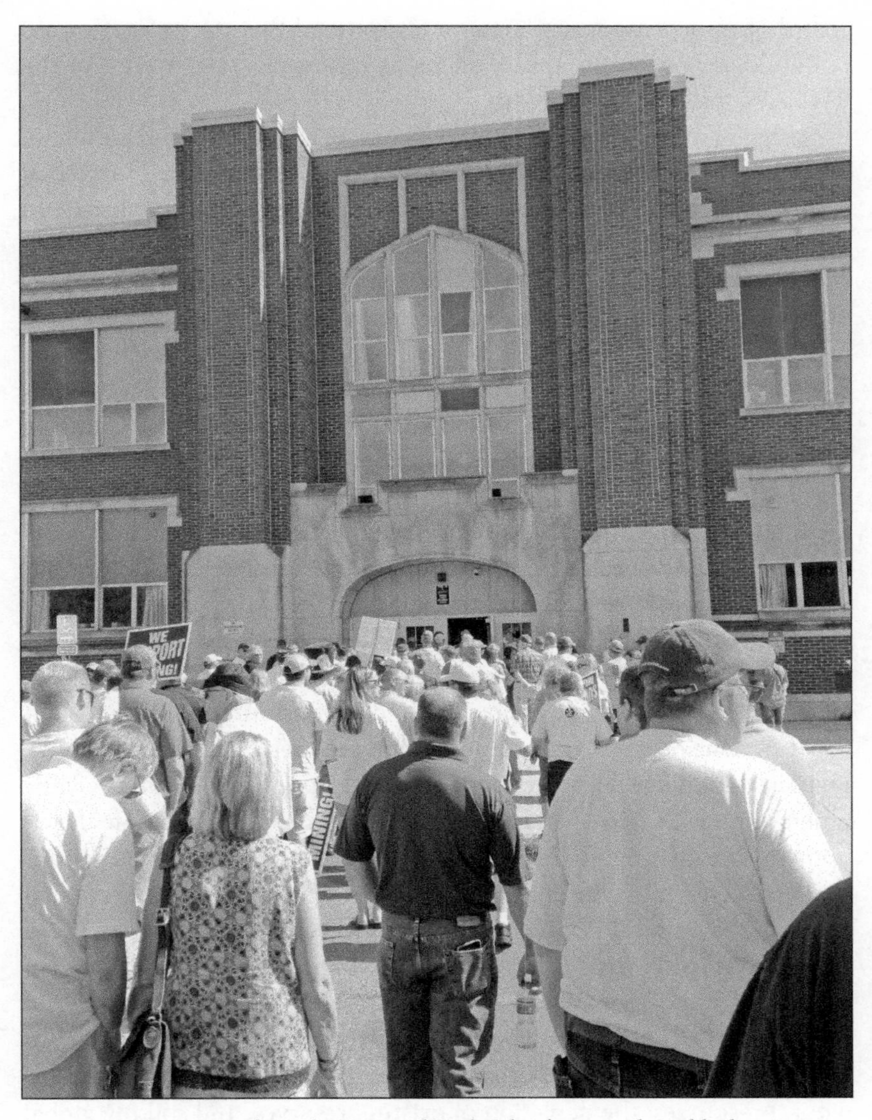

Mining supporters march to Ely Memorial High School to attend a public hearing on the Twin Metals mining project. (Photo by Erik Kojola)

crowd of mine supporters. Opponents claimed that the project would pollute the clean water and damage the wilderness experience of the BWCAW, thus hurting tourism.

Struggles over how to use natural resources and public land are all but inevitable, because these decisions are not simply narrow environmental policy issues but debates over identity, morals, the future, and justice. In this book, I explore how such conflicts reveal the cultural, class, gender, and racial politics of resource extraction through a case study of how different white communities respond to proposed copper-nickel mines in Minnesota's Iron Range. The biggest markers of culture and economy "up north" (in local parlance, roughly the entire area of Minnesota north of the Twin Cities and its suburbs) fall into contestation: recreation in the Land of 10,000 Lakes and mining in the Iron Range. Here, "enduring conflicts" between environmental protection and industrial development go beyond simple jobs-versus-the-environment explanations and belie typical portrayals of resistance or passive acceptance of hazardous industries.[1] These are complex conflicts over the meaning of place, collective memories, and future imaginaries, all of which are tinged by class, whiteness, masculinity, and the context of settler colonialism and global capitalism. There is active opposition and support for new industry, but there are tensions and ambiguities within and between these positions. Politicians on the left are divided, with some opposing new mines while others align with right-wing politicians and industry to promote development. Meanwhile, there are tensions among environmental groups and between white conservationists and Indigenous groups over what places and communities to prioritize for protection.

This real-world fight over mining development in rural midwestern towns and cities resonates with growing conflicts in the US and around the world as people grapple with how to live in the ecological and social devastations brought by capitalist extraction.[2] Rising demand for natural resources, the depletion of existing reserves, and spiking global commodity prices are driving a boom in mining.[3] Creating new locations, types, and methods of extraction often poses risks to public health, biodiversity, clean water, and the acceleration of climate change, threatening working-class, racialized, and Indigenous communities in particular.[4] At the same time, these projects provide profits for multinational corporations and come with the prospect of new jobs and state revenue in what are often rural regions weathering economic and social dislocation.[5] In the US, the Republican Donald Trump administration accelerated mining and industrial projects with controversial decisions about the Pebble Mine in Alaska, uranium mining near the Grand Canyon, and coal mining in the Bears Ears National Monument in Utah that were protested by environmental groups and Native American tribes.[6] Initial signs from the Democratic Joe Biden administration suggest that some of those actions may be reversed, although not without resistance from industry and aligned politicians. Yet Biden and many other Democrats are also supportive of domestic mining and oil and gas extraction in the name of resource independence and supplying materials for the green energy economy, although with some limits in the name of environmental protection.

Minnesota has no copper, nickel, or other nonferrous-metal mines, which carry new risks (see chapter 2 for details on the mining process).[7] Iron mines, instead, dominate, giving the Iron Range its moniker since the late twentieth century. The region is one of the largest global producers of iron, and massive open-pit mines mark the landscape. At the Hill Annex mine, which closed in 1978 and is now a state park, visitors can take a bus tour through the old, rusted buildings and between the large piles of orangish-red waste rock and gaze over the mine pit that is now flooded with water. Yet some mines are still operating, such as the Hibbing Taconite mine, which has been operating since the 1920s and now offers visitors a viewing deck to scan the horizon over an eight-mile-wide pit and watch massive trucks, as tall as two-story houses, that look like specks hauling ore in the distance. For a better sense of scale, you can walk up to a retired ore-hauling truck outside the visitors' center; at six feet tall, I barely reached the midway point of the huge rubber tires. Today, mining companies, investors, and local politicians envision a resource boom, with more trucks excavating metals from below the surface of northeastern Minnesota, predicated on the extraction of previously unprofitable low-grade but supposedly "world-class" copper and nickel reserves via technologies touted as safe and economical.

Certainly, economic and demographic indicators suggest there may be widespread support for new mining: the Iron Range and the broader Arrowhead region of northeastern Minnesota, like other rural and

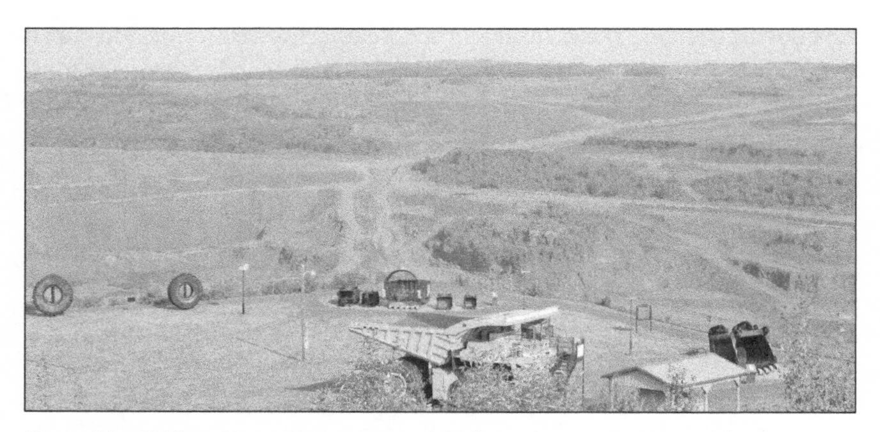

View of the Hibbing Taconite Mine, one of the largest open-pit mines in the US. (Photo by Erik Kojola)

mining regions, is dealing with a lack of good jobs and a shrinking and aging population. Once-bustling downtowns have boarded-up windows and for-sale signs on storefronts, and residents watch their grocery stores close and local schools consolidate due to a lack of students. Politically, the area has shifted to the right. Iron Range residents face what the sociologist and environmental justice scholar-activist Robert Bullard calls "economic blackmail" as they seemingly have to choose between polluting mining jobs or a lack of decent jobs.[8] People also feel that their way of life, collective history, and community identity are under threat. Thus, predominantly working class and white residents and unions, alongside local politicians and industry groups, have mobilized to promote copper-nickel mining as a way to restore their communal pride and prosperity. Mine supporters use a discourse of *extractive populism* to assert that mining development is a way to protect the nation and the people—coded as white, working class, and rural—against outside threats from urban elites, federal bureaucrats, and foreign, often racialized, countries and to reassert a moral economy based on family-supporting wages for white, masculine labor.

So, where is the conflict and opposition? Copper-nickel mines carry greater environmental risks than existing iron mines do and threaten Minnesota's famed sky-blue waters. The lakes in northern Minnesota draw people from across the state and country for vacations and weekend getaways to fish for walleye and to canoe in remote areas where the only sounds are the soft splash of paddles and the eerie call of loons. This has propelled copper-nickel mining into one of the most contentious political issues in the state. Organized opposition from environmental, conservation, and Indigenous groups has tied up proposals in long regulatory, legal, and political processes with uncertain outcomes. Government agencies have been inundated with public input, as state records were shattered for the amount of comments on an environmental impact assessment. I attended many hearings in packed auditoriums and convention centers, where hundreds and thousands of people wearing "Save the Boundary Waters" and "Mining Supports Us" stickers sat for hours listening to remarks lobbed at government officials.

Yet opponents are not unified and differ over what areas should be prioritized for protection from new, risky development: less-populated wilderness areas or more-populated areas already facing legacies of industrial pollution. When the mines are sited near Minnesota's popular (and protected) BWCAW, there has been strong opposition from conservationists and outdoor recreation groups and companies—largely

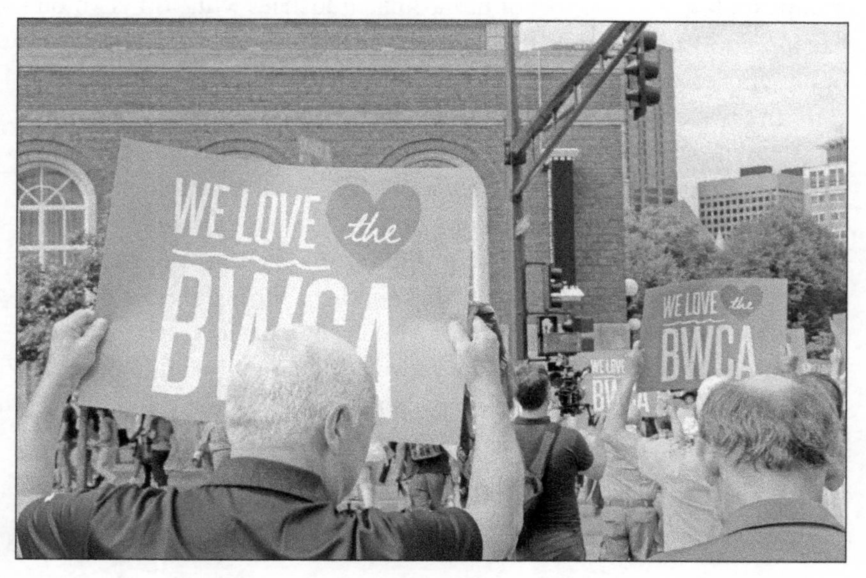

Mining opponents march to a public hearing in St. Paul, Minnesota. (Photo by Erik Kojola)

middle-class and white constituencies from urban and suburban areas. They claim the mantra of *wilderness populism* to make an ethical, political, and emotional assertion that this is public land for the enjoyment of all Americans, not for private profits from destructive and polluting mining practices. Other environmental groups and Native American tribes have prioritized opposing a mine that would add further pollution burdens to downstream and Indigenous communities and threaten treaty rights to hunt, fish, and gather. They emphasize concerns about public health and clean water. These differences reflect long-standing tensions in the US environmental movement over prioritizing wilderness conservation and recreation or human health and pollution.[9] These are tensions between mainstream environmental groups with predominantly middle-class and white members and environmental justice groups with more working-class, people of color, and Indigenous members.

Throughout this book, I examine how contentious politics and mobilization over mining and environmental conservation are shaped by three interrelated issues tied to political-economy and cultural dynamics of class, whiteness, masculinity, and place. First, I consider why some groups mobilize in support of hazardous industries while others mobilize in opposition. I explicitly focus on the largely white supporters and opponents of mining to understand how whiteness and differences in class and place shape relationships to land. How do different groups understand the risks of industrial projects and see development as bringing justice or injustice? Material benefits are a common explanation for why people support hazardous development, and material harms (including pollution and health effects) are posited as the driver of opposition.[10] Each explanation is incomplete. What happens, for instance, if both the economic benefits and environmental risks of a project are uncertain? Why and how people mobilize for and against extractive and other hazardous industries are also a cultural, ideological, emotional, and political process shaped by power.[11] Therefore, I explore how people's cultural frameworks—the lenses through which they understand and describe the world, which vary across intersections of place, class, race, and gender—influence perceptions of risk and justice.

Second, I examine how different groups of white people across rural-urban and class divides engage in environmental politics. What strategies do activists, corporations, and politicians use to negotiate environmental decision-making and mobilize support? I study different stakeholders including rural residents, unions, environmental organizations, conservation and outdoor recreation groups, and government and industry elites to understand how different cultural frameworks lead to different positions and political strategies. Previous research tends to focus on one side, but I explore the divergences and similarities across different groups. I am especially interested in how various actors assert authenticity and legitimacy as they frame issues. How do emotional appeals to collective history and place-based identities mobilize action? Which appeals are regarded as *authentic*? In particular, how do different sides assert populist claims of standing up for "the people"?

Third, I situate contemporary mining controversies in Minnesota across time by examining regional histories, collective memories, and hopes for the future and across space by assessing how local dynamics are interconnected with national and transnational forces. This offers insights into political-economic processes shaping rural and industrial regions across the US and the political realignments of white, working-class, and rural constituencies. I examine how mining struggles are tied to a conservative shift in the historically democratic Iron Range. How have conservative politicians used populist and racist appeals to the symbols of mining, natural resources, and rural places to both wield and accrue power? This helps clarify the social and political-economic forces that have swept right-wing populists into office, like Donald Trump in 2016, and that continue to upend the Republican Party. Global commodities markets and transnational corporations are driving resource production in peripheral rural regions like the Iron Range but are also encountering local-level friction related to the particular geological, ecological, cultural, and historical context, particularly concern for wilderness and clean water.[12]

Proposed Copper-Nickel Mining in Northeastern Minnesota

Minnesota's Iron Range is a social and geological region that spans over one hundred miles from the small city of Grand Rapids, Minnesota, in the southwest to the town of Ely, Minnesota, in the northeast. It's within the broader Arrowhead region that encompasses four counties in the northeastern corner of the state up to the shores of Lake Superior and includes the midsized city of Duluth. The region's iron-ore deposits have been mined since the late nineteenth century, spurring European colonization and settlement and capital investment (which depended on and required the displacement and genocide of Ojibwe, Dakota, and other Indigenous peoples). By the 1940s and '50s, the Iron Range was a principal source of raw materials for the US steel industry, busily building US cities and automobiles.[13] Towns and small cities developed around the mines with bustling downtowns where miners drank coffee at diners before their shifts and drank beer after work at the many bars, and people shopped for bratwurst and Finnish rye bread at the local butchers and bakeries. Mining royalties were used to build ornate high schools and townhall buildings. Yet later shifts in the global steel industry, overseas competition, and increased mechanization left the area contending with unemployment, poverty, and population loss.[14] Today, many of those storefronts have closed, and buildings are going into disrepair. The landscape still carries the marks of mining: "lakes" that are flooded mine pits where crystal-blue waters are surrounded by reddish-orange waste rock, mining memorial sites with bronze plaques and old excavators, and the occasional rumble of detonations at the mines still digging out iron ore. Mining heritage has even been turned into tourism: on the Mesabi Trail, you can walk or bike along 145 miles of path that weaves between forests of spruce, aspen, and jack pine, small towns, and two-hundred-foot-tall mounds of mine tailings. Tall metal fences with "Danger" and "Private Property" signs make sure you do not stumble onto company property or into an active mine site.

The geology of northern Minnesota attracted a resurgence of interest from global capital in the early 2000s, when international copper and nickel prices were at historic highs. A slate of multinational mining companies began exploring projects in the region's Duluth Complex—a geological formation thought to contain one of the world's largest reserves of copper and nickel along with other base and precious metals.[15] Technologies have made extracting and processing ores more efficient, raising the potential profitability of mining even low-grade ores.[16] The two most advanced and contested proposals are PolyMet's NorthMet project and Twin Metals' Minnesota project (both are small Canadian mining companies but are financed and owned by Glencore and

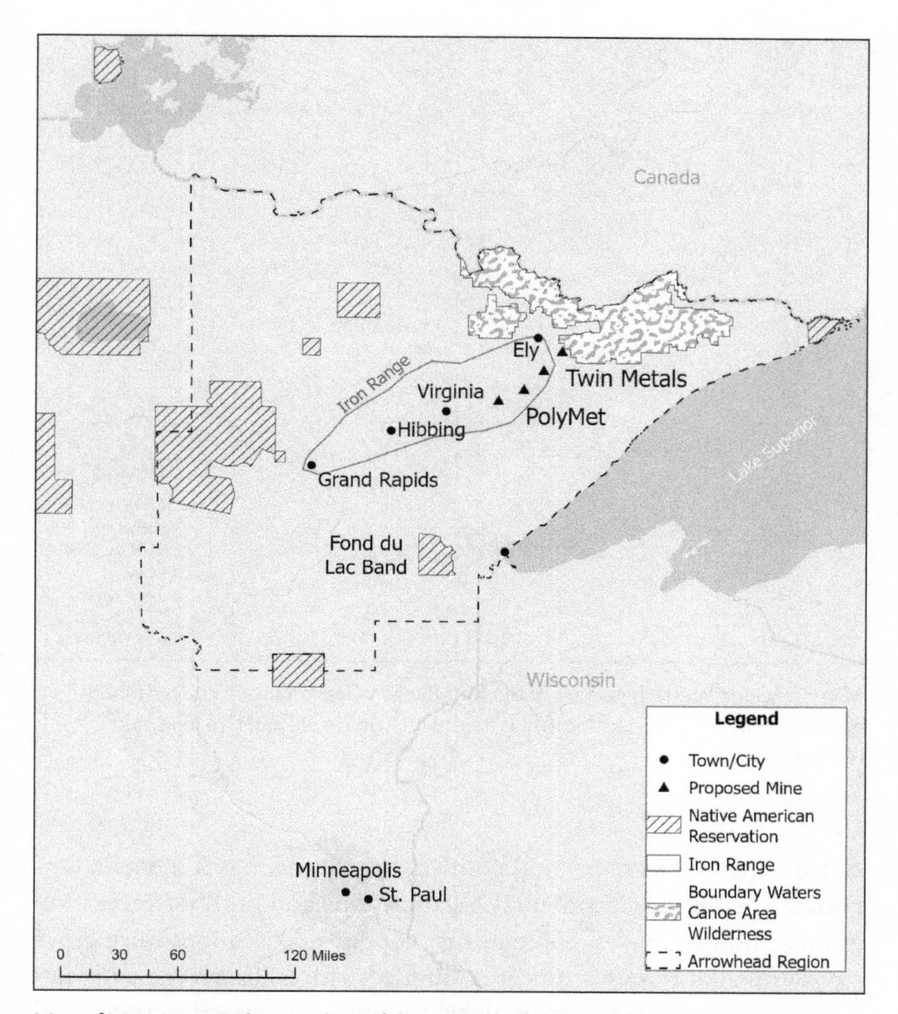

Map of Minnesota with an outline of the counties that constitute the Arrowhead region and a circle around the Iron Range. (Created by Erik Kojola and Cristopher Gianakopoulos)

Antofagasta, a pair of large, multinational mining corporations); at least three other companies are also conducting exploration.

What began as relatively uncontroversial bureaucratic and technical decisions about new mining in a mining region grew into a highly contested political issue. As exploratory studies and emerging scientific knowledge highlight the environmental risks of the mines, public

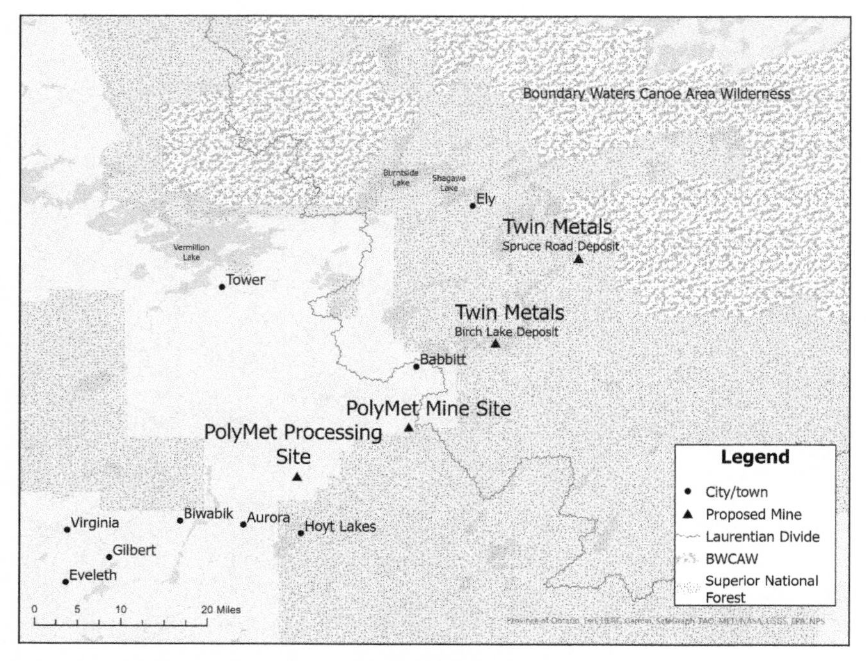

Map of the northeastern portion of the Iron Range where proposed copper-nickel mines and the BWCAW are located. (Created by Erik Kojola and Cristopher Gianakopoulos)

concern, as well as social and political opposition, has fomented. Opponents, led by environmental organizations and outdoor recreation groups and businesses, contend that copper-nickel mines raise grave environmental risks for this area studded with lakes, rivers, and wetlands. The process of copper-nickel mining involves extracting small amounts of valuable metals, leaving behind large amounts of waste rock suffused with sulfide minerals. When those sulfides are exposed to air and water, they create hazardous sulfuric acid—what is called acid mine drainage—potentially leaching heavy metals and damaging aquatic ecosystems. Twin Metals' mine has drawn especially widespread opposition on these grounds since it would abut the BWCAW, one of the country's most visited wilderness recreation areas, where it is possible to canoe for hundreds of miles through undeveloped land without hearing a motor vehicle or seeing a road.

Mine proponents, including mining corporations, industry groups, construction and mining unions, local politicians, and Iron Range residents, have led a countermobilization. To promote development and build political and social support for mining, they argue that the new mines would create much-needed jobs and revenue while leveraging the latest technologies to keep the environment clean. Still, there are tensions within the region. Brandon, whom I got to know during my fieldwork while spending time at the weekly farmers' market and microroaster coffeeshop in Ely, embodied the complexities around mining. He was from Ely, and his grandfather had worked in the iron mines; but Brandon thought the new copper-nickel mines were too risky and a bad idea. His position created tension with some family members, who saw mining as their way of life and key to the future.

Over fifteen years down the line, neither PolyMet's nor Twin Metals' projects are certain and remain embroiled in legal and political battles.[17] Divergent court rulings and shifting political winds have left the projects in legal and political limbo, while the vagaries of global commodities markets and international finance may ultimately determine their fate.

An Emblematic and Unique Region

Environmental politics are often local, so research must address the ways people understand the particular places in which environmental conflicts unfold and the environments in which they live, work, and play.[18] Even in contemporary global capitalism, place and the local level remain relevant; economic processes operate across transnational, national, and local scales and occur within concrete social, ecological, and political contexts.[19] The Iron Range thus provides a rich but understudied site to examine interconnected local and global dynamics of mining and the cultural class politics of resource extraction and conservation.

The region is emblematic of rural extractive regions in the US. Like Appalachia and the Powder River Basin of Montana, the Iron Range is geographically isolated, predominantly white, economically depressed, and dominated by a powerful mining industry.[20] The economy here reflects what the environmental and rural sociologist William Freudenburg has termed "addictive economies"—regions dominated by resource extraction that become hooked on the industry despite its environmental, social, and economic costs (amid instabilities of boom-and-bust resource markets).[21] Extractive regions often have a strong community identity, a double-edged sword that means there is both a strong sense of solidarity and an insularity and cultural skepticism toward "outsiders."[22] Being an "Iron Ranger" in Minnesota is a strong, place-based identity rooted in the region's history of mining and white European ethnic traditions developed from earlier generations of eastern European, Italian, Scandinavian, and Finnish immigrants.

The tradition of immigration, mining labor, and outdoor recreation also makes the Iron Range distinct in important ways. The region has a unique history of leftist politics, an avid outdoors culture, and relatively robust state environmental regulations.[23] Its labor struggles are long-standing, led by the mostly male mine workers who fought mine bosses to organize strong unions and improve working conditions.[24] In the early twentieth century, there were socialist newspapers published in Finnish, active Communist Party chapters, and support for the anarcho-syndicalist Industrial Workers of the World. Unions, although much less radical, continue to be an important political and social institution in the region. This labor and immigrant history is why the Iron Range has been a Democratic stronghold and a key part of the governing coalition with progressive farmers and urban voters that established Minnesota as a Democratic stronghold.

Northern Minnesota is also known for its sky-blue waters and white-barked birch trees. Two million acres of boreal forests with stands of spruce, fir, aspen, and birch trees cover northern Minnesota, including the BWCAW, and provide rich habitat for deer, moose, gray wolves, and lynx. The lakes dotting the landscape attract people seeking to fish for walleye and lake sturgeon and listen to the call of loons echoing across the still waters at dusk. Residents from across the state talk about "going up north" to get away on weekends and vacations to lake cabins, ice huts, and campsites. During my fieldwork in Ely, I would often strap a kayak to the top of my car at the end of the day and drive to one of the many nearby public boat launches to spend an hour paddling before the sunset, watching birds diving and fish jumping to feed on insects.

Iron Rangers are passionate about the outdoors, whether its deer hunting in the fall, ice fishing on frozen lakes in the winter, or riding all-terrain vehicles (ATVs) in the summer. Many gas stations in the

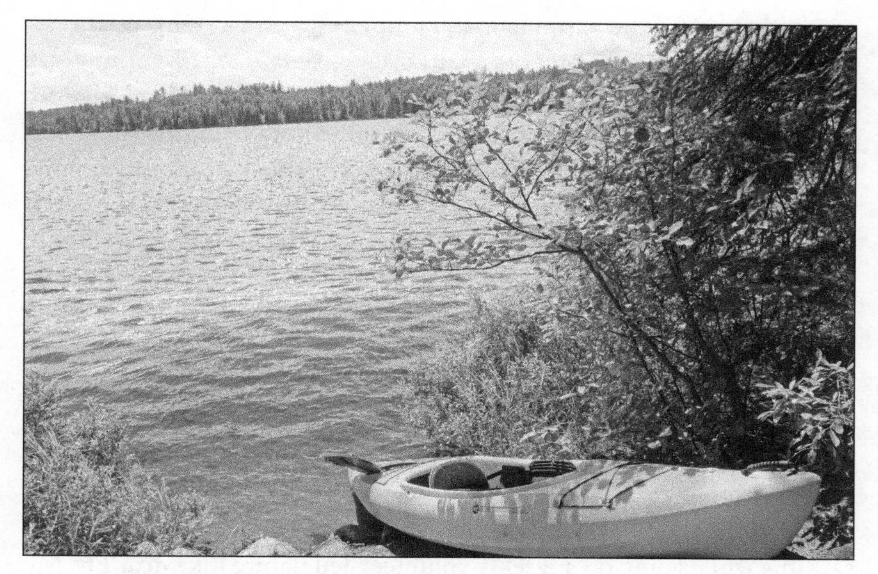

A lake near Ely, Minnesota, popular for boating and fishing. (Photo by Erik Kojola)

region sell live bait, and much of my small talk with people at cafes and shops in Ely centered around recommendations for fishing spots and canoeing routes. One morning while I was sitting at the counter of a long-standing diner drinking a mug of light-brown coffee and reading the *Ely Echo*, two men in their seventies sat next to me. They knew the waitresses by their first names, and the waitresses brought them their orders without asking. They were discussing whether they had seen any fawns in the woods yet—a sign for the upcoming hunting season—and asked me if I had, which began a conversation about wildlife in the area. The conversation shifted as they went on to lament the restrictions on using motor vehicles in the BWCAW and environmentalists who were simply opposed to "everything."

In the eastern and northern parts of the Iron Range that are near the BWCAW, people are relocating to live near the outdoors during retirement or to work remotely or in the tourism industry. Yet, unlike parts of the West, like Montana, Colorado, and Oregon, where former mining and logging towns have recently begun transforming and gentrifying into tourist and retirement destinations, the lakes and forests of northern Minnesota have attracted people seeking recreation and solace for generations. And the extreme inequalities between working-class residents and wealthy newcomers seen in places like Jackson, Wyoming, are not as extreme in northern Minnesota, where poverty among longtime residents is not as high and the newcomers are not the ultrawealthy and global elite.[25] It was out of the ordinary when someone rich and famous came to the area. For example, I heard a rumor that Bill Gates visited to look at property in the region, which had created local buzz—supposedly he decided not to buy after coming in the winter. The progressive political history and popularity of outdoor recreation also contribute to Minnesota having relatively strong environmental protections and a large environmental movement, particularly compared to other states with large extractive industries, like West Virginia or Arizona.[26]

My case-study site, the Iron Range, thus belies some of the patterns found in other rural and extractive regions and some of the common assumptions about US rural conservatism and anti-environmentalism. I saw this while going on a weekly volunteer-led nature hike near Ely. My fellow hikers were from all walks of life, including a woman in her sixties from Ely, a mother and her two children who lived in a nearby town, a couple from Florida who were architects and owned a lake cabin in the area, and an elderly couple who spent their summers as volunteer hosts at a state-park campsite. Local, working-class residents were out on a hike through the dense forests and marshy fields listening to birds and learning about ecosystems alongside upper-class professionals visiting from out of state wearing Patagonia clothing and toting high-powered binoculars.

Culture, Place, and Power in Environmental Politics

In what follows, I draw on environmental sociology, political ecology, cultural sociology, and social movement studies to consider the dynamics of power, political-economy, and culture in one community's fight over a new, risky form of mining. In this book, I examine how different groups understand and mobilize around extractive development and the racial, gender, and class meanings of land and natural resources that help to explain why decisions about resource extraction in rural mining areas have consequences for contemporary politics and social movements.

Common explanations for resistance to or acceptance of hazardous industries are the evidence for pollution and material benefits to accrue from a given project. Scientific data documenting the effects of pollution can make a problem visible, but objective evidence does not necessarily drive responses to hazardous industries.[27] People may support nearby industry even when there is evidence of pollution harming human health; people may oppose industry despite a lack of scientific evidence proving health risks. Why people accept or oppose polluting industries is also tied to their material dependence on the industry for their livelihoods. In mining communities, working-class residents rely on the jobs and revenue and often lack economic alternatives, so they can be more willing to accept environmental risks than those who live farther away as well as middle- and upper-class locals whose livelihoods are not reliant on the industry.[28] Yet experiences with the ill health effects from industrial pollution can create critical interpretations of mining and spur resistance to industry.[29]

Environmental sociologists and political ecologists argue that reactions to polluting industrial projects do not fit neat categories of acceptance or opposition. Rather, how people make sense of these projects is a complex cultural and ideological process laden with power that goes well beyond scientific data and material interests.[30] Power operates through ideologies, culture, language, and everyday interactions, such that people consent to domination and come to see the status quo as common sense, while resistance can also occur in subtle ways and through overt political action. Stephanie Malin's research on how rural western communities respond to nearby uranium mining shows that economic dependence, collective identities, and attachments to place help round out our understanding of people's reactions to risky industrial development. Malin points out that those who have been most impacted by a dirty industry may also be the most likely to support the industry's renewal. The sociologist Kari Norgaard's examination of climate change denial emphasizes that people's perceptions of environmental risks are a collective process shaped by cultural frameworks and emotions.[31] Working-class and rural residents of mining towns are not simply duped by corporations into a false class consciousness, yet industrial pollution can become normalized, even celebrated, while expansion of hazardous industries is seen as necessary for future well-being and a way to reaffirm a moral economy when collective identities are tied to industry.[32] The sociologist Rebecca Scott's analysis of the cultural, racial, and gender politics of mountaintop removal coal mining in Appalachia in her book *Removing Mountains: Extracting Nature and Identity in the Appalachian Coalfields* uncovers the ways that land and resource struggles are about space, place, identity, and emotion. Scott troubles common categories of class, race, worker, and environmentalist to show the complex and ambiguous ways that people understand an environmentally destructive practice and reconcile love of place and community identities tied to coal.

In the Iron Range case, we see a blend of resistance and acceptance that comes into focus when we look at the different class and regional cultural frameworks. People evaluate industrial practices and relate to the nonhuman environment through their cultural frameworks, which are schemata used to make sense of the world and include shared beliefs, values, language, and norms that provide scripts for interpreting social problems.[33] While there are dominant and national cultural schemas, people also have agency in interpreting and reconfiguring them.[34] Cultural frameworks also vary across social locations, identities, and geographies. Importantly, how these frameworks are constructed, and used, is a process of struggle and power. They shape what is taken for granted and what is imagined as possible. Throughout the book, I emphasize the links between class, place, masculinity, and whiteness that are integral to people's worldviews and identities.[35]

Land and conservation politics are struggles over place, but place is not just a physical location. Places are made through the ways that people relate to a geographic location and assign it cultural meanings.[36] This means that "place" depends on people's lived experiences, daily interactions, and collective memories—shared stories about the past that help make sense of the present and direct future-oriented action.[37] Place, in this way, can tie people to a broader community and serve as a foundation to their cultural framework.[38] While rural places are small in population and geographically isolated, it is their social, not only physical, boundaries that make them culturally and politically meaningful. Rural places in the US have a powerful identity tied to being a cohesive moral community with shared values and ways of life, often defined in contrast to supposedly dangerous, fast-paced, and alienating cities.[39]

The collective meaning of place, particularly in rural places dominated with a single industry, is also connected to labor as well as class, race, and gender. The environmental sociologists Shannon Bell and Richard York's research in West Virginia coal-mining regions describes how community economic identities linked to industry are constructed and maintained through politics, the media, popular culture, and appeals to masculinity and patriotism that help sustain the industry's legitimacy despite pollution and dwindling jobs.[40]

Social class and its intersections with other social locations and systems of domination are fundamental in shaping people's relationships to place and their cultural frameworks.[41] Throughout the book, I explore the cultural, discursive, and symbolic aspects of how social class becomes meaningful for people, rather than just people's structural class positions.[42] I draw on cultural theories of class to analyze how class shapes people's worldviews, social practices, daily lives, and the symbolic boundaries constructed around communities.[43] Class distinctions are tied to various forms of social and cultural capital that intersect with gender, race, place, sexuality, and nationality.[44] Class is also spatial and produced within places. Living in rural or urban places and working in different types of jobs inform people's habitus—embodied practices, language, and cultural tastes that carry different status meanings.[45] People who interact with nonhuman nature through recreation may view the landscape as one of aesthetics and leisure, while workers who interact with nonhuman nature through labor may see that same place as an industrial landscape.[46]

In the US, class is inseparable from race and interconnected systems of white supremacy, race-based chattel slavery, and settler colonialism.[47] Whiteness is a constructed racial category that grants privileges and benefits to those who are racialized as white. Workers and unions have long been coded as white and male, even though the US labor force and labor movement have increasing numbers of women, people of color, and immigrants.[48] Historically, some unions have worked to secure exclusive benefits for their white male members, particularly in extractive and industrial industries, and blocked people of color and women from getting these privileged "breadwinner" jobs.[49] Thus, the class locations of Iron Rangers are intertwined with the dominance of mining work by white men and its association with hegemonic masculinity.[50] Throughout the book, I emphasize how the connections between place-based, class, gender, and racial identities cultivate social action, particularly through people's emotional ties to memories and future imaginaries.

Land and natural resources in the US are also tied to racism, settler colonialism, and patriarchy. Displacement of Indigenous people to enable settlement of white Europeans and extraction of value from nonhuman nature was justified by racist and masculine claims of "civilizing" savage people and wild lands. Ecofeminist scholars, such as Caroline Merchant, Val Plumwood, and Greta Gaard, argue that systems of hierarchy and the domination of nonhuman nature are legitimized by interlocking dualisms that position society versus nature, masculinity versus femininity, white versus nonwhite, and rationality versus emotion.[51] Men are on the dominant side of these dualisms, linked to civilization, science, and strength, and thus in a position to control nature and women. Hegemonic masculinity often valorizes domination of nature, physical strength, risky and dirty work, and being a breadwinner—symbolized in blue-collar male workers like miners.[52] The interconnected ideologies of patriarchy, settler colonialism, and whiteness imbue white settlers, particularly men, with a belief that they have a right to turn land into private property and extract value from nonhuman nature.

These logics continue to shape anti-environmental, anti-government, and militia movements. For example, the 2016 armed takeover, led by Ammon Bundy, of the Malheur National Wildlife Refuge in Oregon was largely about white men claiming their "right" to property and using violence to do so.[53] The feminist political ecologist Cara Daggett describes "petro-masculinity" as a discourse linking fossil fuels materially, emotionally, and culturally to systems of white patriarchy and hypermasculinity that rely on intensive fossil fuel consumption.[54] Support for fossil fuels, which is strongest among white conservative men, becomes a way to protect hegemonic masculinity threatened by ecological and environmental crises as well as shifting gender norms. This form of hypermasculinity is also at work in support for other extractive industries and anti-environmentalism. Yet hegemonic masculinity and extractivist discourses are also flexible. In response to widespread concerns about environmentalism and sustainability, industry and its supporters have constructed an ecomodern masculinity that appeals to technology, economic growth, and scientific expertise to present industry as clean and dedicated to protecting the environment.[55]

Environmentalism and conservation are also imbued with masculine and racist ideas about white Europeans needing to save and tame nature through modernization and science while creating protected wild places for adventure and recreation.[56] This leads to solutions from traditionally male domains of science and engineering and a paternalistic approach to protecting a feminized nature.[57] The influential environmental historian William Cronon argues that the idea of wilderness as a place untrammeled by humans was constructed in the US by erasing Indigenous people's use of the land for millennia and creating a false division between human society and nonhuman nature.[58] Still, environmentalism can also challenge hegemonic masculinity. Formative research by R. W. Connell, a prominent sociologist of gender and masculinity, explored how men's involvement in the environmental movement in Australia reshaped their understandings and practices of masculinity, reconfiguring hegemonic masculinity at least at a personal level.[59]

In bringing together these different fields, my approach builds on social movement scholars who have examined the role of collective identities and emotions in how and why people mobilize politically.[60] Social movements try to frame issues—identifying, explaining, and assigning blame—in ways that are interpreted as legitimate, authentic, and truthful according to people's cultural frameworks in order to mobilize social action.[61] Particularly important are the affective meanings of place and collective memories that are powerful in influencing how and why people engage in social mobilization to defend a place, whether by reinforcing or resisting dominant social systems.[62] Defense of place can be progressive, such as Black communities demanding environmental justice by resisting dumping of toxic waste, or reactionary, such as white ranchers taking up arms against the federal government to defend their free access to ostensibly shared public land.[63] Residents of rural extractive regions may identify their community and sense of place with industry, internalizing a sense that often exploitative and polluting industries are inevitable and naturalized as part of the place while also seeing threats to industry as a threat to their collective identity.[64] The dominance of extractive industries can be challenged by competing narratives that position industrial development as risky and a threat to meanings of place tied to outdoor recreation and experiences of nonhuman nature.[65]

Overview of Findings and Contributions

Throughout the book, I show that decisions about developing polluting, extractive industries engender such enduring and passionate conflicts because they are political, economic, and cultural struggles. Collective identities and memories of place are animated by masculinity, class, and whiteness, which inform how different groups perceive risks and frame their positions in order to assert legitimacy. The particular historical, social, and political context of northern Minnesota influences how future extraction is understood and framed, but in ways shaped by broader discourses such as tropes about upper-class environmentalists and backward rural "rednecks." Mining and wilderness areas both carry powerful symbolic meanings related to "the nation" and "the people"—which are tied to whiteness in the US—that are made emotionally meaningful through populist appeals to romantic nostalgia and hopeful imaginaries.

First, my approach connects environmental, political, and cultural sociology to show how emotions and identities shape perceptions of environmental issues and framing strategies used by social movements, politicians, and corporations. The emotional meanings of place motivate mobilization around contentious environmental issues and inform perceptions of environmental justice in ways that both challenge and reinforce dominant socionatural relations. That is, class and regional cultural frameworks lead to divergent assessments of risk and justice on the Iron Range and to competing assertions to speak for the place. I show the importance of emotions in discursive strategies used by both pro-environment and pro-development coalitions and how the passionate responses to land and natural resource use matter for broader politics.[66] Understanding these dynamics is important for building bridges across class and region and creating coalitions to promote socioecological justice. My analysis provides insights for environmental groups on how to frame issues in ways that connect with rural and working-class people.

Second, I offer insights into the ways that populism is a flexible rhetorical style and discourse taken up by environmental and anti-environmental movements.[67] Populism often involves appeals to "the people" and claims of defending them against a threat (for instance, foreign powers, wealthy corporations, immigrants, and racialized others).[68] Populists of all stripes construct a sense of threat or crisis and propose its solution—empowering the people and returning to a nostalgic past—but they differ in defining "the people" and characterizing their hoped-for restoration.[69] Left-wing populist claims can promote inclusive visions that challenge the status quo (mobilizing "the people" against those who hold power), while right-wing and authoritarian movements tend to invoke "the people" as a way to inhibit coalition building by appealing to a more exclusive, racialized, and gendered vision of ideal citizens.[70] In northern Minnesota, groups use competing populist frames to claim that they are defending the people, the land, and the nation—which is seen as intrinsically white in the US—against threats and powerful interests in order to assert cultural authority.

Specifically, residents and community leaders leverage a discourse of *extractive populism* to assert that rural people have the morally inflected right to determine how their backyard is used, rather than supposed outside elites, who are portrayed as seeing the area as their playground. Extractive populism promises to renew masculinity by putting men back to work doing physically demanding jobs and restoring heteronormative families with men in their place as breadwinners. It also appeals to defending the nation against foreign threats by securing resource independence. Copper-nickel backers in Minnesota also use an ecomodern masculine discourse, claiming that companies and regulators can be trusted since new technologies will keep their cherished lakes and forests clean. Iron Rangers argue they will not despoil the place they know deeply through everyday experiences and labor. Instead, they assert that mining development advances justice by allowing locals to extract value from the land and maintain their moral economy—the norms that govern economic activity and the moral obligations between workers, capital, and the state—based around male breadwinners and corporate taxes supporting local services.[71]

Yet some mining opponents respond with a discourse of what I call *wilderness populism*: the land belongs to the people, and the broader public (not only locals) has a right to influence decision-making and ensure corporate and government accountability for protecting the environment. Opponents *also* claim to know the place intimately. They profess their love for the natural beauty and recreation opportunities offered by the Iron Range, and they draw attention to scientific research documenting the risks of resource extraction. The opposition, comprising primarily urban and middle-class people, views mining as too risky for a cherished place, as a harbinger of *in*justice in which private companies profit while degrading public land and water for future generations. This frames technocratic environmental policy debates about science in a more authentic, legitimate, and emotionally resonate way. Yet opponents still work within the dominant discursive and political context and also use appeals to scientific expertise and data.

Third, my analysis challenges assumptions about environmentalism and class. All groups claim to care for the environment and claim that data and research is on their side—indicative of how discourses about environmentalism, science, and sustainability have become dominant. The "sides" in the copper-nickel-mining debate do not align neatly with expected categories. There are all sorts of tensions within the alliances promoting and opposing mining. In particular, the different locations of proposed mines—one in the watershed of a wilderness area and the other in a watershed already contaminated by industry—lead to different reactions and strategies among opponents. Conservation and outdoor-recreation groups have different priorities than do environmental groups and tribal organizations working on broader environmental issues and environmental justice. Some conservation and recreation groups prioritize efforts to stop the Twin Metals mine near a beloved wilderness area, while tacitly accepting PolyMet's proposed mine closer to population centers and the Fond du Lac reservation. Other environmentalists are focused on the PolyMet project since it would affect larger downstream communities in a watershed already impacted by years of industry and mining. All this reflects long-standing race, class, and political tensions saturating the US environmental movement.[72]

Many working-class Iron Range residents are concerned about protecting clean water but reconcile it with support for new mines by placing trust in corporate claims about safety and remembering iron mining as having a clean history. In other moments, the very same supporters critique the very same companies and corporate powers. It is important to disentangle the actions of nearby residents and industry workers, who are not simply pawns of industry but do operate within dominant ideologies and political-economic conditions. Understandably, there are tensions within the unlikely alliance of mine supporters, including union members, libertarian and state's rights activists, Democrats, and right-wing Republicans. Smaller, grassroots pro-mining groups are connected to broader right-wing networks and use social media to share information and amplify attacks on the federal government. Yet other Iron Range residents and leaders as well as unions reject this broader pro-corporate and neoliberal agenda. They support progressive economic and social policies alongside mining development. Unlike the sociologist Loka Ashwood's book *For-Profit Democracy: Why the Government Is Losing the Trust of Rural America*, which depicts a state legitimacy crisis in rural Georgia, the government, particularly at the state level, retains some legitimacy in Minnesota for many residents—pro-mining groups argue that the rigorous regulatory process should be followed since it can ensure that mining is safe. Environmentalists—rather than government—are seen as the primary threat to the local moral economy.

Fourth, I show that decisions about extractive industries in rural areas have expansive political consequences. Conflicts over mining are a key symbolic issue that has contributed to the twin rise of right-wing politics and anti-environmentalism, combined so potently in *extractive populism*. Class, gender, racial, and cultural frames go some distance in explaining why appeals to defend a rural, white, and masculine mining way of life are so powerful and resonant, helping to maintain the mining industry's and political leaders' legitimacy by conferring them with the coveted imprimatur of authenticity. Nostalgic appeals to a romantic past in response to a sense of lost social status are a common feature of right-wing movements in the US and Europe that attracts white, working-class, and rural people, particularly men.[73] Rising global precarity and uneven development, which creates spaces of disinvestment, devastation, and ruin, creates a context in which appeals to nostalgia and hope are powerful mobilizing frames. I add an analysis of the environment, emotions, and place-based identities to recent research on right-wing populism among white, rural, and working-class people, using my case study to flesh out the cultural politics of mining and the social and political consequences of economic dislocation.[74] Promises to restore the mining heyday in the context of economic dislocation offer a sense of hope while strengthening the white nation and hegemonic masculinity by reaffirming the moral worth of rural communities and male mine workers, who often feel disparaged by mainstream culture and urbanites.[75]

Methodology

The book is based on a multimethod qualitative case study, drawn from the collection of in-depth interviews, document analysis, and ethnographic observation conducted primarily from 2015 through 2017. In my Iron Range case study, I am able to observe how, why, and to what effect political and regulatory decisions were made regarding copper-nickel mining; how diverse actors from different social locations mobilize and interact in these struggles; and how individuals explain their positions. Multiple forms of data allow me to develop deeper insights into social dynamics through observations of real-world interactions, conversations with people, and close reading of textual sources.[76] My research is focused on environmental and pro-development groups and activists closely involved with the copper-nickel-mining issue; thus, I do not attempt to capture broad public opinion or to determine relative levels of support and opposition to mining or Indigenous views on mining.

My ethnographic research for this project came in two components. From 2014 through 2017, I observed public events, including all the meetings held by government agencies around the state about the copper-nickel-mining projects, such as public comment sessions on environmental impact statements and presentations about the regulatory review process. Concurrently, I attended events organized by environmental groups in Minneapolis–St. Paul, from lectures and presentations to fund-raisers, film screenings, and rallies, as well as mining-industry conferences. All these events helped me understand how state officials talk about the projects, how people engage in bureaucratic decision-making, and how different groups are mobilizing for and against the proposed mines.

In 2017, I undertook a summer of fieldwork in the Iron Range town of Ely, Minnesota (supplemented with several shorter trips to the region to gain further data). I learned about the physical and cultural landscape of the town and region, gaining insight into the nuances of the social and geographic context through my daily interactions and experiences.

TABLE I.1. Categories and Number of Interviews

Type of interviewee	Number interviewed
Environmentalists	32
Experts and scientists	21
Industry representatives	3
Small business owners	7
Politicians	6
Pro-mining activists	4
Government agency staff	7
Residents of Iron Range	17
Union representatives	3
Tribal representatives	1
Total	101

Note: I classify someone as an Iron Range resident if they are not actively involved in pro-mining or environmental groups and could be supportive or opposed to copper-nickel mining. Environmentalists, government agency staff, and small business owners may also live in the Iron Range, but I classify them according to their primary role in relationship to the copper-nickel-mining controversy.

I went to social and cultural events, visited local museums and mining memorials, attended meetings of environmental and pro-mining groups, and spent time in public spaces such as cafes and the grocery store. I created relationships and developed trust and credibility by spending time where residents socialized, including a weekly luncheon and lecture organized by a group of retirees and weekly nature walks led by volunteer naturalists.

I conducted 101 in-depth semistructured interviews from spring 2015 to summer 2017 with representatives of different stakeholder groups, including environmental and conservation organizations, labor unions, businesses and industry groups, Iron Range residents, politicians, government agencies, and scientists, to capture a diversity of perspectives (see table I.1 for a complete list). I categorize people on the basis of their jobs and active participation in groups involved with copper-nickel mining. To gain breadth, I spoke to a wide range of groups and organizations, from statewide to grassroots, as well as people in different positions within organizations; at one environmental organization, for example, I interviewed everyone from senior leaders to young field organizers.

To find participants, I used a mix of purposive and referral sampling.[77] I identified key leaders of organizations through websites and press coverage, and sought interviewees who were highly involved with copper-nickel-mining issues. I also met people at events, such as volunteers with an environmental group at a summer festival, and used referrals to make new connections and identify informal community leaders.[78] Networking and making personal connections was essential for developing relationships with Iron Range residents, union members, and grassroots environmental activists who could not be identified through public information and for whom establishing my credibility was essential for them to be comfortable sitting for a formal interview. Interviews lasted from forty-five minutes to two hours and were semistructured conversations guided by pertinent topics and key questions.[79]

I analyze data from newspaper articles, public documents, and organizational materials to assess public debates, discourse, and framing as well as to create timelines of events.[80] Newspaper data are drawn from the *Star Tribune*, Minnesota's largest and most circulated newspaper, and three popular regional newspapers, the *Duluth News Tribune*, the *Mesabi Daily News*, and the *Timberjay*. I collected articles from 1999, when PolyMet began exploration, through January 2017, when key decisions were reached on both projects. National news coverage and online sources provided further context but were not part of my systematic textual analysis.

My archival data also include organizational documents (such as websites, social media, and newsletters) from environmental and pro-mining groups and mining companies; these data concern how groups frame issues, create policy positions, and develop advocacy tactics.[81] Public documents, such as environmental impact statements and company annual reports, are used to create a record of how and when official decisions are reached and to provide information on the scientific, engineering, and legal issues. They are supplemented by industry data from investor analysis and demographic, economic, and voting data from public sources.

Ethics and Reflexivity

Knowledge is never completely objective, absolute, or neutral. It is inherently embedded in power and social relations.[82] We particularly owe a debt to feminist theory, which argues that knowledge is embodied and produced from somewhere, in ways shaped by people's social positions and politics.[83] My political views, biography, and social location as a white, settler, middle-class, heterosexual, and cisgender man shape everything from the questions I ask to the conclusions I reach.

My interest in this case study is motivated by my biography and political commitments, namely, my family connections to northern Minnesota and involvement in both the labor and environmental movements. Though I was raised on the East Coast, my father, who spent his career working with unions on occupational health and safety issues, is descended from Finnish immigrants who settled in Hibbing, Minnesota, an Iron Range town perhaps best known as Bob Dylan's hometown. I grew up hearing stories about and even visiting the "Range," not least because my mother is also from northern Minnesota, born into a family active in the labor movement and progressive politics in the major iron-shipping port of Duluth. My own experiences working in a labor union before graduate school and my continued involvement in labor and environmental organizations, coupled with my roots in northeastern Minnesota, give me unique insights into the worldviews of some of those who are duking it out over copper-nickel mining on the Iron Range. They have also left gaps.

Navigating power dynamics is particularly challenging in fieldwork, more so when the researcher comes from a different social location than participants and further yet when it is a more privileged position than some participants. Thus, being young, white, middle class, and male shaped my interactions and how people perceived me in ways that opened up some networks and created other challenges. My social position helped me establish connections with white men who were small business owners, former and current mine workers, union members, and middle-class environmentalists—these participants would often chat with me about masculine hobbies like fishing, canoeing, and hunting. It also created skepticism among those residents and workers who suspected I was, as a young graduate student from "the city," an environmentalist uniformly opposed to mining. For example, when a male retiree in Hoyt Lakes, Minnesota, suggested that I attend his weekday-morning coffee group at the town's diner, the others—mostly retired miners—vetoed his invitation. They were worried about what I would do with the information and how I would represent their views. A male researcher may have also seemed more threatening. For example, male interviewees often asserted their masculinity, like telling me about their physically difficult and dangerous work in mining or prowess in repairing old cars, which may have been an attempt to establish some dominance, especially if they perceived me as being in a higher socioeconomic status position. Still, most people, especially when I was able to explain my project and my desire to understand a range of perspectives, were welcoming. In this, my Finnish surname and family connections to Hibbing were useful; participants often wanted to chat about my family history and make jokes about Finnish culture. Some of the same aspects of my social position—being white, middle class, male, and connected to the university—were helpful in opening access among experts, policy makers, and environmentalists, in that they bolstered perceptions of my legitimacy. Environmentalists, especially the college-educated urbanites, saw our shared cultural milieu and that I am an academic studying environmental issues and assumed that I was "on their side."

I was careful not to become an active participant in any organizations or to take a public stance on the proposed mines. I aimed to access all sides, though I am aware that my apparent neutrality came at the expense of some measure of in-depth knowledge and meaningful relationships. Personally, I am skeptical of the copper-nickel-mining proposals, especially claims made by these multinational corporations about safety and job creation. I think there is abundant evidence that the projects could bring pollution and that there would be limited long-term benefits to community members. Yet I also witnessed moments when environmentalists exaggerated their claims and overlooked the perspectives of Iron Rangers and the struggles facing workers and rural communities.

In part, my detachment also means that Indigenous perspectives were not central in my research. This is an intentional decision based on my belief that ethical research with Indigenous communities requires collaboration and long-term relationships of trust and accountability. Building the relationships to do research with Indigenous communities and tribes requires participatory and community-based scholarship that would have been incompatible with also interviewing businesses, conservative politicians, unions, and mainstream environmentalists. I chose to focus on building trust to interview rural residents and pro-mining groups, even as I recognize that my choice serves to amplify only the perspectives of white settlers like myself and leaves out Indigenous experiences. In the book, I address settler colonialism and point to silences in the dominant discourse that overlook Indigenous perspectives; I also draw on public statements made by tribes and Indigenous organizations as well as a formal interview with an intertribal resource-management organization and interactions with tribal resource managers during work on a different university-tribal collaborative research project. There is a wealth of writing from Indigenous scholars and activists and settler allies that elucidates Indigenous environmentalism, cultural and spiritual worldviews, and political struggles.[84]

Outline of the Book

I begin in chapter 1 with background on the social, political, economic, and environmental history of the Iron Range, setting the stage for my exploration of collective identities and memories as well as contemporary mining struggles. The region is shaped by global political-economic and ideological processes ranging from European colonization and Indigenous dispossession to shifts in global markets and development of mining technologies. It is also a resource-rich area home to long-standing conflicts over resource extraction and environmental conservation, particularly around protecting the Boundary Waters and the creation of the protected conservation area known as the Boundary Waters Canoe Area Wilderness.

Chapter 2 turns to the copper-nickel-mining proposals at hand. I situate these proposals within political and economic conditions—particularly the global copper-mining industry—and the geochemical and geographic distinctions between copper-nickel and iron mining that have made the former contentious in an area dominated by the latter. This is followed by the stories of the PolyMet and Twin Metals proposals, highlighting stakeholders, legal and regulatory issues, and key turning points in the projects' progressions.

The mining controversy is also rooted in collective identity and meanings of place, as I consider in chapter 3. Divergent class and regional cultural frameworks help people make sense of copper-nickel mining in ways that see both opponents and proponents mobilizing to defend ideas like who counts as a "local," who has the right to speak for the land, and who will best protect the environment. My analysis suggests that Iron Range mining proponents see this region as an industrial mining landscape, while opponents view the same region as a wilderness and recreation landscape that all people have a right to use, setting up the dynamics of extractive and wilderness populism discourses that are further explored in chapter 5.

But before we get there, chapter 4 considers the role of time and emotions in the contested politics of mining. Different groups' collective memories and future imaginaries, that is, also figure into the establishment of these ideological worldviews. Proponents hope new proposals will renew the mining past to create a prosperous but "traditional" future; opponents see new extractive projects as a threat to their collective memories of outdoor recreation and the ability of future generations to use the place in "traditional" ways. I show how the affective meanings of the past and future are powerful in mobilizing political action, regardless of its direction.

Chapter 5 shifts to the political implications of conflicts over copper-nickel mining and explores how mining has become a symbolic site of contention in wider rural-urban and class divides. Mining supporters use a discourse of what I term *extractive populism* to rally support of rural, white, and working-class residents, effecting, in part, a rightward political swing for the historically leftist Iron Range. I argue that place-based and class identities linked to mining are important in how right-wing populist movements use mining to create an image of authenticity and emotional appeals to defending "the people."

I conclude by reflecting on the key themes and lessons from my case study for national politics and social movements. Arguments over copper-nickel mining are about the past, present, and future and divergent visions of a good life. Overcoming seemingly intractable conflicts between the environment and the economy, and bridging class and regional divides, will necessitate engaged and carefully tempered discourse to create solutions to address the socioenvironmental crises created by global capitalism and extractivism. Just transition policies are needed that get rural and industrial communities out of the jobs blackmail bind while providing culturally meaningful types of work and reaffirming people's collective identities.

1

A Contested Place

Legacies of Extraction and Conservation in the Iron Range

Geological and ecological processes have created a place rich in minerals and timber and a unique landscape of dense forests and interconnected lakes that is popular for outdoor recreation in the Arrowhead of northeastern Minnesota. This landscape has shaped the region's history of settler colonialism, extractive capitalism, and wilderness conservation, its contemporary culture and political economy. A seemingly isolated and rural place at the northern edge of the US, with long, harsh winters, the Iron Range has been interconnected with global political-economic processes from the development of European colonial fur trading to today's global supply networks and metal and minerals markets. This landscape sets the terms of the debate when it comes to struggles over copper-nickel mining and environmental protection.

In subsequent chapters, I will turn to those vigorous debates. First, we need to dig into the region's history, highlighting the displacement of Indigenous peoples, labor organizing, and conflicts over resource extraction and outdoor recreation focused on the Boundary Waters Canoe Area Wilderness. All these inform the collective memories, future imaginaries, and place-based identities that people mobilize as they make sense of—and take sides on—the copper-nickel-mining proposals that animate, invigorate, and divide Minnesotans today.

Brief History of the Minnesota Iron Range

The Iron Range within the Arrowhead region is defined socially by its strong cultural identity and collective history of mining, and it is defined geologically by a series of mineral ranges rich in iron, copper, and nickel. Home to about 150,000 people, the Iron Range is in the far northeastern corner of the state and spans over one hundred miles from Grand Rapids, Minnesota, in the southwest to Ely, Minnesota, in the northeast, which sits on the edge of the BWCAW and the border of Canada. The region is around two hundred miles from the Twin Cities metro region and roughly thirty miles from Duluth, Minnesota—the state's fourth-largest city, which is a major shipping hub on the shores of Lake Superior, where trains dump iron ore into massive barge ships, providing ready access to global markets. The region includes several geological deposits, including three iron deposits (the Mesabi, Vermillion, and Cuyuna ranges) and the Duluth Complex, which yields copper, nickel, and platinum group elements (PGE) as well as small amounts of gold, silver, and other precious metals. The Duluth Complex, which the current mining proposals hope to tap, is a formation of volcanic and sedimentary rock formed 1.8 billion years ago, in the Precambrian era. There, the base metals of copper, nickel, and zinc have combined with sulfur to create sulfide-ore minerals, among them the large stores of low-grade copper and nickel sulfide ore that have aroused renewed industry interest in the twenty-first century.[1]

Extractive Capitalism, Dispossession, and Labor Struggles

European colonists and multinational corporations have long sought profits in the lands that constitute what is now called Minnesota. This land, however, like the rest of North America (the landmass known to some Indigenous peoples as Turtle Island), is the ancestral and current homeland of Native American peoples and hundreds of different tribal nations. The Anishinaabe, a cultural and linguistic group that includes Ojibwe, Potawatomi, and Algonquin, and the Oceti Sakowin (or Sioux, which includes Lakota and Dakota peoples), have lived here for millennia. Because extractive capitalism and settler colonialism depend on the displacement of Indigenous peoples like the Anishinaabe, the environmental justice scholars Lisa Park and David Pellow call resource extraction a form of racial domination and environmental injustice.[2] Without the theft of land and genocidal violence, rationalized through ideologies of racial inferiority, the conversion of the Iron Range into a capitalist's playground never could have happened. In Minnesota, as across the US, colonizers, entrepreneurs, and the federal government deployed violence, coercion, and legal measures to remove Indigenous inhabitants, acquire their land, and make way for extractive capitalism.[3]

The US government signed treaties with Ojibwe, Potawatomi, Menominee, Ho-Chunk, and Dakota tribes to acquire the land in the Upper Midwest that is now the states of Minnesota, Wisconsin, and Michigan.[4] The treaty process was undertaken according to rules and terms that were not set by or often fully understood by tribes, which were pressured and coerced into negotiations. Indigenous scholars describe how tribes understood treaties as ceremonial exchanges meant as the basis for lasting relationships of reciprocity and mutual goodwill.[5] The US government, on the other hand, saw treaties as a way to acquire land and resources and also to pacify Indigenous communities through subjugation. The treaty and relocation process pushed tribes onto cramped reservations of marginal and relatively unproductive lands; private companies and white settlers acquired thousands of acres of prized, productive land (often made so by generations of Indigenous stewardship).[6] The 1854 Treaty of La Pointe was signed by Lake Superior Chippewa (an anglicized term for Ojibwe) bands, including the Fond du Lac, Grand Portage, and Boise Forte Bands from Minnesota; the L'Anse, Vieux de Sert, and Ontonagon Bands from Michigan; the La Pointe, Lac du Flambeau, and Lac Court Oreilles from Wisconsin; and the Mississippi River Chippewa bands from Minnesota. The 1854 Treaty covered more than two million acres in northern Minnesota, including the current-day Iron Range and BWCAW. It also created the Fond du Lac, Grand Portage, and Boise Forte reservations in Minnesota as well as several others in Wisconsin and Michigan.[7] The tribes negotiated for payments as well as continued access to hunt, fish, and gather in the ceded territory, beyond the boundaries of the new reservations.

Displacement and the transformation of land into private property opened up corporate investments. As the US rapidly industrialized in the late nineteenth century into the twentieth, extractive industries sought to convert the region's abundant forests and mineral-rich soils into salable goods, quickly transforming the region's physical and social landscapes. The logging industry expanded in the mid-1800s, spurring growth of the newly formed state of Minnesota. When, by the 1900s, the pine and spruce forests of northern Minnesota had been largely depleted and production began to slow, the lumber mills began to close. By 1930, most were already gone.[8] The reduced industry limped along, and as of 2016, some five hundred people in Minnesota's Arrowhead remained employed in forestry and logging. That number is expected to decline further over the next decade.[9]

In the meantime, mining rose to replace logging as the region's major industry. It, too, brought large-scale development and migration. In the 1860s, prospectors spurred a short-lived gold rush near the current town of Tower, Minnesota; they uncovered little gold, but large iron deposits were revealed.[10] These became valuable in the 1870s and 1880s, when increased demand for steel, advancements in the steel-making process, improvements in rail transportation, and legal changes to federal mineral rights made iron mining profitable.[11] In 1883, Minnesota's first commercial iron mine was established in Tower. By the 1890s, several underground mines in the area, including Ely, were shipping iron ore on newly built railroads to the ports in Duluth, where it was shipped to steel factories around the Midwest.[12] The iron-mining industry expanded westward, where geological conditions enabled larger and more profitable open-pit mines at the close of the century.

The Iron Range, a regional designation encompassing all three iron complexes in the area, was soon among the world's largest iron producers, and it was integral to US industrialization as it fed steel mills and factories across the country.[13] Industrialists, including John D. Rockefeller, Andrew Carnegie, and J. P. Morgan, invested heavily to build new mines and to consolidate small mining companies into large, vertically integrated companies, like US Steel, which owned mines in Minnesota and steel foundries throughout the Midwest.[14] Mineworkers' late nineteenth-century settlements and camps grew into permanent towns and cities, and by 1920, the region had a permanent population of around one hundred thousand people—the vast majority of whom were non-Indigenous.[15] Jobs in the mines attracted thousands of European immigrants, largely from Finland, Slovenia, Croatia, Italy, and other parts of southern and eastern Europe. In 1910, nearly 80 percent of the region's population were first-generation immigrants.[16]

An economy dominated by a single mining industry brings booms and busts due to unstable global prices, technological changes, geopolitics, and resource depletion. This means that the fortunes of the Iron Range have always been at the mercy of national and global economic swings. Downturns like the Great Depression mean decreased production and high unemployment (a measure that hit 70 percent in the Iron Range during the 1930s).[17] Periods of economic growth, such as World War I and World War II, were a boon, as US demand for planes, automobiles, and kitchen appliances kicked steel production (and, in turn, iron mining) into high gear.

Geological factors and technological changes have also shaped the region's history. The region struggled in the 1940s and 1950s. High-grade natural iron-ore deposits were being depleted, and so iron-mining production slowed and jobs fell away. However, development of new technologies and methods to process and refine low-grade iron deposits, called taconite, brought a new boom era in the 1960s.[18] More than a dozen taconite plants breathed life back into the iron-mining industry, but booms and busts, unemployment, population loss, and a lack of economic diversification continued to challenge the region.[19] Automation and mechanization allowed companies to increase production with fewer workers, and so ore production continued to rise as employment in Minnesota's iron mines dropped.[20] Massive, open-pit taconite mines additionally raised the scale and speed of extraction, using trucks, explosives, and other machinery but fewer and fewer workers. A downturn in the international steel market and a drop in the price of steel in the 1980s proved that the taconite industry—and the region—was just as vulnerable as high-grade iron mining and forestry to the uncertainties and fluctuations of the global capitalist economy.[21]

Initially, work in the iron mines was dangerous and low paid, and the companies vehemently resisted unionization. It took decades of long and brutal organizing efforts as well as changes in national labor law for mine workers to create the strong unions that transformed mining into a good job with decent pay, benefits, and safer working conditions.[22] These fights unfolded through the early to mid-twentieth century, and companies fought back with violence and coercive anti-union tactics. The first major strike, in 1907, failed; the companies broke the strike without significantly changing working conditions.[23] A decade later, workers walked off the job at several mines. They sparked the 1916 Mesabi Range strike, supported by the anarcho-syndicalist Industrial Workers of the World (IWW). In the long struggle that ensued, several miners were killed, and many more were arrested. Workers gained minor concessions toward improving pay and conditions, but the companies resisted recognizing the workers' union. Through the 1920s, mine bosses stifled organizing through control, repression, and paternalism.[24] Another wave of union activism, in the 1930s, was led by the Congress of Industrial Organizations (CIO) and achieved another set of modest successes, yet weak national labor laws, company opposition, and the onset of World War II again stymied efforts to establish unions in the mines of the Iron Range.[25]

In the World War II and postwar era, mine workers finally established unions and gained collective bargaining rights across the region. Their success was related to broader political-economic conditions including a tight labor market, high demand for steel, and New Deal–era changes to labor law, all of which advantaged workers. The United Steel Workers (USW) led these renewed organizing efforts in the 1940s. It had won recognition at many of the mines by 1943, and, by the 1950s, all the Iron Range mines were unionized.[26] The USW and the mining companies, buoyed by a profitable era of high industrial demand and consumer confidence, entered a period of relative peace, a detente in which workers gained better pay and safer working conditions.[27]

Today, histories of labor fights and radical politics are remembered on the Iron Range, though they are often presented as a relic of the past rather than an ongoing, perpetually relevant struggle. This depoliticizes contemporary labor issues and enables mining companies to frame themselves as good neighbors who provide decent jobs and give back to the community—silencing how high wages, health insurance, and safe working conditions were gained through struggle. When I visited the Minnesota Discovery Center, a large regional museum and tourist center, in 2017, it was to view a special exhibition on the 1916 Mesabi Range strike. I was surprised at its positive portrayal of leftist politics and workers' militant actions; the exhibit told a story of corporations using violence against workers while communists and anarchists helped organize the workers. Still, the *radical past* that the exhibit celebrated was utterly disconnected from the contemporary moment. The Mesabi Range strike exhibit stood alongside mining-company-sponsored exhibits celebrating the innovative iron industry and the ingenuity of modern mining technologies. There was no mention of ongoing labor struggles, unemployment, population loss, or health and safety concerns surrounding the mines—helping contemporary companies maintain their rosy public image while ignoring the forces of globalization and neoliberalism that have created economic woes in the Iron Range and towns and cities across the rural US.[28] Class and labor strife was laid out for the public as important, necessary, and settled in the distant, sepia-toned past.

The legacies of class struggle, union organizing, and radical politics embraced by largely European immigrant mine workers all contributed to making the Iron Range a stronghold of leftist politics, and they continue to shape the region's political culture. Many of the early Finnish, eastern European, and Italian immigrants to the Iron Range were active in anarchist, communist, and socialist politics in Europe. They brought their political ideas and tactics with them to northern Minnesota, where socialist halls and leftist, foreign-language newspapers became common.[29] As workers clashed with mining companies, their collective anger at enormously wealthy, absentee owners coalesced into a distinctly working-class, anti-corporate ethos and identity, mobilized at the ballot box.

The region has historically been represented by progressive politicians at the local, state, and national levels. Its voters have consistently picked candidates endorsed by the Democratic Farmer Labor (DFL) Party—its very name an enduring symbol of the state's progressive politics and urban-rural voting alliances, adopted when the Democratic and socialist-leaning Farmer-Labor parties merged in 1944.[30] Iron Range towns like Hibbing were notorious for electing leftist leaders who demanded high taxes and large royalties from mining companies. Over time, it became a given that the Iron Range voted for the DFL. Aaron Brown, a cultural commentator and community-college instructor in Hibbing, sums up this sentiment by writing, "the Iron Range has elected Democrats as reliably as the orbit of the moon."[31]

The DFL's power is crucially tied to the strength of Iron Range unions, whose politically active members have historically formed the backbone of the party's regional support, membership, and leadership—although union influence and member allegiance to the DFL have waned in recent years. Active and unified political participation also contributes to the Iron Range's powerful influence on statewide politics. The conventional wisdom is that all roads to the Minnesota State Capitol run through the Iron Range.

Iron Ranger Identity: Hard Work and European Ethnicity

The histories of mining and immigration and living in an isolated, rural place have created a tight-knit community and strong collective identity: "Iron Rangers." It is constructed through the population's sense of self-reliance, pride, and community solidarity, all necessary to its continued survival in this isolated place, with its harsh climate and poor soils and its boom-and-bust economy dominated by unstable extractive industries.[32] Brown notes that, in this place-based culture, "Most folks committed to living here long term know that they may have to dig up some other way of life if their current gig runs out, as most gigs eventually do. That creates resourcefulness and a strong work ethic."[33]

European ethnicity and immigration histories are inextricable from what it means to be an Iron Ranger, too. Though immigration flows had significantly slowed by the 1920s and 1930s, European ethnic identities have remained strong as generations live and die in this insular region. Thriving cultural traditions and practices account for the Finnish saunas common to Iron Range homes and the polka music and dancing that enliven local bars and community halls.[34] The historian Mary Lou Nemanic argues that Iron Rangers maintained customs from Europe far longer than much of the rest of the US, resisting "melting-pot" Americanization to create and carry forward a unique form of US regional identity.[35] My own casual conversations in towns like Ely confirmed the continued salience of European ethnicity as longtime residents deduced each other's ethnic heritage from their surnames and their families' past addresses—neighborhoods and towns once segregated by nationality still provided reliable clues. Older residents recognized my own surname as Finnish, smiling as they jokingly corrected my Americanized pronunciation and declared me "Suomi" (the Finnish word for Finland).

The flip side of this passionate Iron Ranger identity and local solidarity is a certain hostility to outsiders.[36] "The area is deeply skeptical of outsiders, but at one time, it housed one of the most diverse immigrant populations in the country," Brown comments.[37] In fact, it was the disparate immigrant groups' need to unite against outside forces that helped them overcome ethnic divisions. Political and union leaders further leveraged insider-versus-outsider framings to consolidate support, initially against East Coast mine bosses and more recently against urban environmentalists.[38]

Today, identifying as an Iron Ranger means coming from a family that has lived in the region for multiple generations and originally immigrated from Europe.[39] The region remains homogeneous—about 92 percent of the population was white as of 2020—because it has not experienced extensive migration or demographic changes.[40] Although Finnish and Italian immigrants were initially racialized as nonwhite and inferior to Anglo-Saxon Protestants, they have become "white." While European ethnic influences can be seen in bakeries selling Slovenian potica cake, white people's ethnic identities are largely what the sociologist of race Mary Waters calls "symbolic ethnicity" that people can choose and use to assert a sense of community without any of the consequences of being racialized as nonwhite.[41]

There are a several Ojibwe reservations in northeastern Minnesota, but only one is partially in the Iron Range: the Boise Forte Band of Chippewa have a small section of their reservation on Lake Vermillion, near the small town of Tower, but the largest section of the reservation is near Nett Lake, west of the Iron Range. The Boise Forte Band has around three thousand enrolled members, but they do not necessarily live on the reservation. Thus, the number of Indigenous people living in the Iron Range is relatively small, although the Ojibwe bands are active in regional environmental issues and natural resource management.

A minor influx of retirees, teleworkers, and small business owners relocating for access to outdoor amenities, especially to towns near the BWCAW, even those who are white and from Minnesota, are excluded from the "Iron Ranger" identity. A fifty-something native of Virginia, Minnesota, Austin moved away from the Iron Range after high school, returning only recently with his Arizona-born wife. Across his dining-room table, Austin told me about the region's social and cultural tensions, remarking that, to be considered an Iron Ranger (in his words, to "have real credit"), you have to "have three generations buried in the cemetery here." Austin's wife was never going to be an Elyite or Iron Ranger.

Nor in this dominant cultural narrative of the true Iron Ranger would the Ojibwe people who have made this place their home for millennia, who continue to live and thrive in and near the region, be included. Settler colonialism and the dispossession of Indigenous peoples are naturalized through white residents' claims to Iron Ranger identity—and to having a unique right to this land. The scholar Chantal Norrgard argues that Indigenous labor and livelihoods based on fishing, hunting, and gathering are typically excluded from discussions about the economy of the Iron Range in order to valorize white, masculine mining labor—as if to confer dignity on the latter requires the erasure of the former.[42]

Struggles over Development and Conservation in the BWCAW

Northeastern Minnesota and areas near the Iron Range are longstanding destinations for outdoor recreation, drawing people from around the state and country to enjoy the crystal-blue waters of lakes scattered throughout the region. Ely, in particular, is a tourist and vacation hub, ranked one of the world's nine best "outdoor towns" by *National Geographic Adventure* magazine in 2016.[43] Bordering the Superior National Forest, the town is known as the "gateway to the Boundary Waters." This beloved dense forest of white and black spruce, fir, birch, aspen, and jack pine, dotted by thousands of interconnected lakes and streams, includes both the BWCAW and Canada's Quetico Provincial Park. Today, the BWCAW alone is the largest federally designated wilderness area east of the Rocky Mountains, a renowned destination for campers, fishing enthusiasts, and boaters eager to explore its twelve hundred miles of canoe routes.[44] It is among the nation's most visited wilderness areas, year after year, and can only be explored on foot or canoe in the spring and summer or by snowshoe, ski, or dogsled in the frigid, snow-covered winters. No motorized vehicles are allowed—not even planes passing overhead.

The creation of this protected area was (and remains) hotly contested. This "embattled wilderness," to borrow a term from the historian David Backes, stirs passionate ideas about how it should be used and by whom.[45] Conservation advocates want the Boundary Waters wholly protected from industrial and commercial uses, while many residents join with mining and logging companies, local politicians, and resort owners in fighting for the area to remain open for "multiple uses," including logging and mining, as well as motorized recreational vehicles.

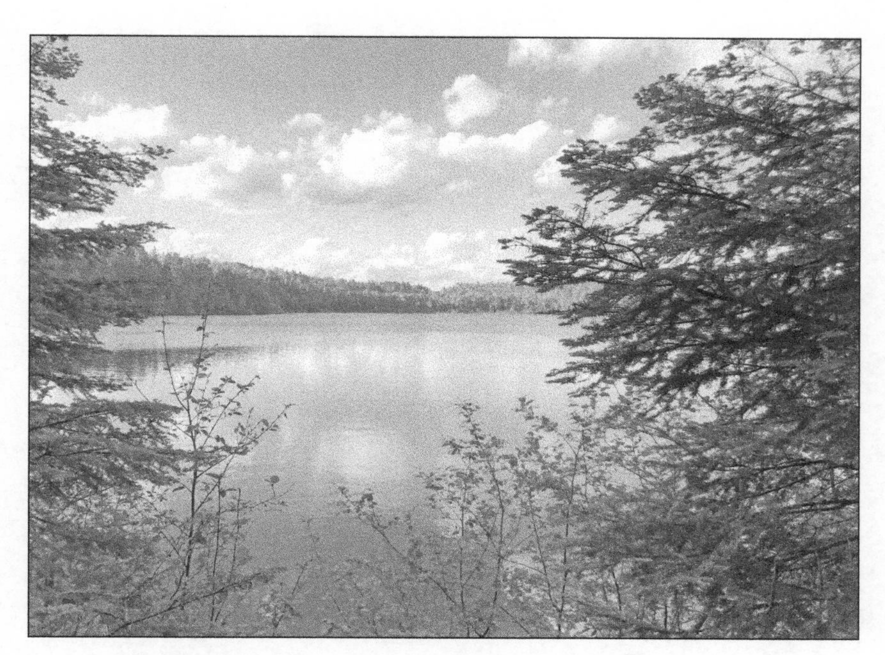

Lake near Ely, Minnesota, outside the BWCAW. (Photo by Erik Kojola)

This is not a new fight: the first settlements in the area housed timber workers, and the first mine sited near Ely, the Chandler Mine, began producing iron in 1888, while the largest, the Pioneer Mine at the edge of downtown Ely, operated until 1967.[46] Recreation, extraction, and conservation regularly collide, and contemporary copper-nickel-mining debates are only the latest iteration of these long-simmering tensions.[47]

Disputes between recreation and extraction are, in fact, common in many regions where mining operations coexist with tourism and service industries connected to natural amenities, as in the mountain towns of Colorado, Utah, and Oregon. Longtime residents whose families came to rural areas to work in mining and logging have different cultures, relationships to the land, and material interests compared to newer residents and vacationers, who are often middle to upper class and move to the area for the natural beauty and outdoor recreation.[48] This can lead to a process of rural gentrification, in which newer, wealthier residents drive up housing prices and living costs, sometimes displacing longer-term, lower-income residents in the process.[49] Tensions also flare

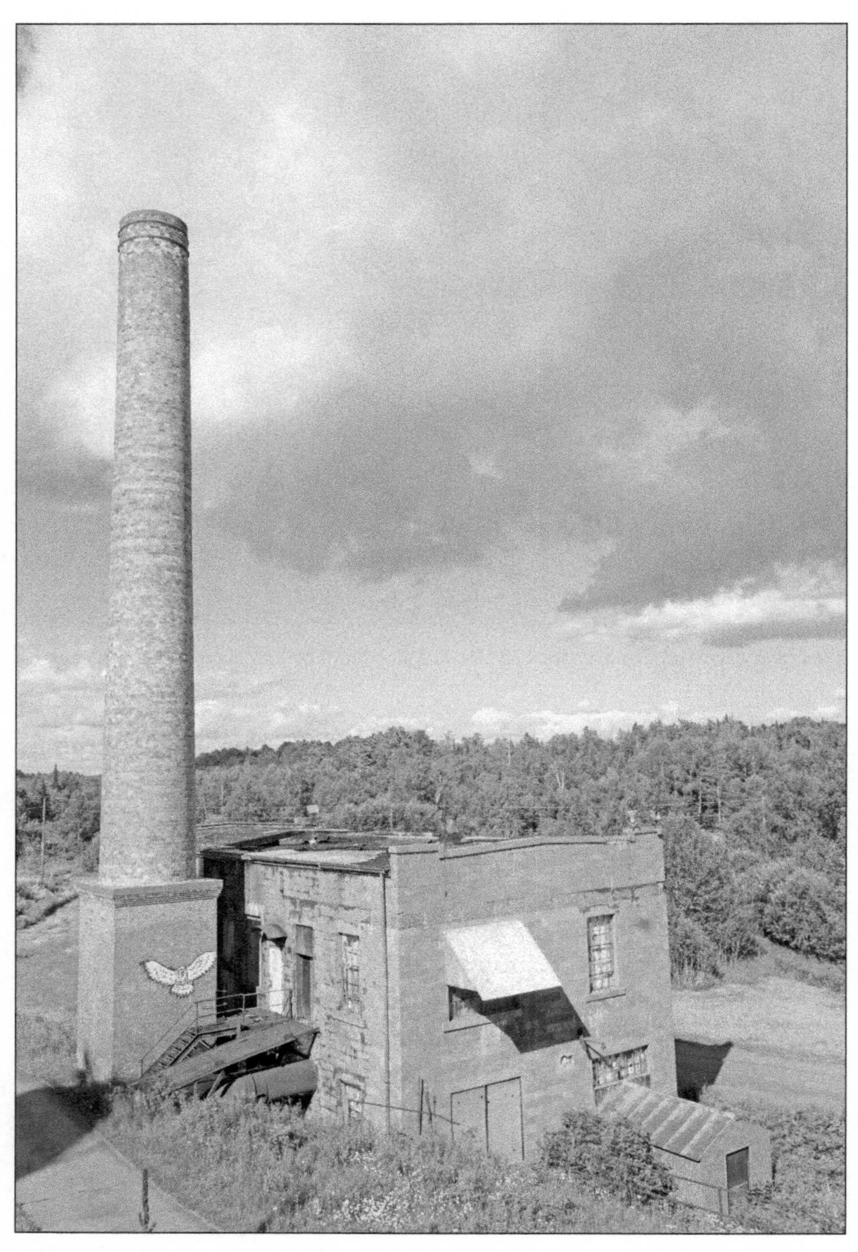

The Pioneer iron mine in Ely, Minnesota, closed in 1967, but remnants remain and now serve as a museum. (Photo by Erik Kojola)

as differing recreation cultures clash. Different people want to experience nonhuman nature differently, and so we see fights between motorized and nonmotorized recreation enthusiasts and between hunters and birders.[50]

In response to the growing conservation movement and concern about rapid industrial development and pollution, the US government took its first steps toward conserving the Boundary Waters in 1902 by excluding five hundred thousand acres of Minnesota land from settlement. Seven years later, Theodore Roosevelt—a proponent of conservation—established the Superior National Forest, which included areas that would eventually become the BWCAW.[51] A roadless area was set aside in 1926 and expanded in 1938 into the million-acre Superior Roadless Primitive Area (SRPA). By the 1940s, Ely was a bustling tourist town, filled with far-flung tourists who came to canoe and fish in the Boundary Waters (there were so many remote, fly-in resorts dotting the region that Ely boasted the largest inland float-plane base in North America).[52]

As conservationists and environmentalists saw planes, motorboats, and hordes of visitors disrupting what they viewed as a quiet and idyllic wilderness experience, potentially even harming the ecosystem, they sought further protections for the Boundary Waters. Over the opposition of some resort owners and tourism companies, the conservationists scored important political victories, notably the 1948 passage of the federal Thye-Blatnik Act, which authorized federal funds for the purchase and demolition of resorts and private cabins in the SRPA. Just a year later, President Harry Truman issued an order prohibiting planes from flying over and landing in the SRPA.[53] A swath of nearby residents grew angry and resentful toward federal interventions and wilderness protections as they were forced to accept paltry compensation for the loss of their private property (although this land was stolen from Indigenous peoples) through federal seizures and saw popular fly-in resorts shuttered.[54]

In the late 1950s and 1960s, conservationists pushing for the creation of a national wilderness system made the Boundary Waters a focal point in their political struggle. At issue were the exact boundaries of the protected area and which activities should be allowed within it. Conservation groups wanted stringent restrictions banning all commercial and industrial activity and any use of motorized vehicles. Many Iron Range politicians and residents opposed the restrictions on logging and mining entirely, and they argued that some areas must remain open to motorboats, ATVs, and snowmobiles. Eventually, federal legislators reached a compromise. The 1964 US Wilderness Act formally created the BWCAW but allowed mining and logging to continue in the adjacent Superior National Forest and carved out exceptions for the use of motorized vehicles on certain designated lakes (they were truly exceptional: the BWCAW remains the only federal wilderness with such allowances).[55] Mineral exploration continued along the edge of the BWCAW, and in the mid-1960s, several copper-nickel mine proposals cropped up, including at some of the same sites that Twin Metals is currently seeking to develop (more on this later in the chapter).

This is not to say that the conflict abated. A pair of federal bills introduced in 1975 and 1976 aimed to further restrict the usage of motor vehicles and logging and mining in and near the BWCAW, triggering years of political fights and social tensions in Ely. Conservation and environmental groups formed statewide and national coalitions to raise public awareness and political support for tougher restrictions on recreational and industrial activities in the BWCAW. Framing motorboats and snowmobiles as pollution threats and affronts to the wilderness experience, these activists tapped into the public's rising environmental concerns. Their opponents, wanting to keep the "multiple use" designation that would allow for conservation, commercial activity, and motorized vehicles, rallied around a portrayal of mining, logging, and motorboat fishing as vital to the region's economy and culture.

Locals in this period staged protests, marches, and rallies, including illegal snowmobile rides through the BWCAW and nailing shut the US Forest Service office near Ely to symbolize that residents were being locked out of their own backyard. Emotional confrontations barely avoided violence in Ely, where one public hearing attracted protestors who hanged an effigy of Sig Olson, a nature writer and conservation leader, outside the US Forest Service office. Staff feared that mob violence could erupt at any moment. Even so, the US Congress defied local opposition, passing the Boundary Waters Canoe Area Wilderness Act in 1978. Along with a ban on mining and logging and further restrictions on motorboats in the BWCAW, the act created a partial buffer zone in which mining was prohibited *outside* the BWCAW.[56] The buffer zone, importantly, left out certain portions of the watershed in which Twin Metals now wants to mine.

The DFL party began to see its urban-rural coalition fray. Party politicians from northeastern Minnesota opposed the BWCAW Act, while DFL politicians from other parts of the state, especially the Twin Cities, were its leading proponents. US Representative Jim Oberstar (MN-DFL), from the Eighth District, described the new wilderness protections as a "Pearl Harbor attack on northern Minnesota."[57] A candidate named Don Fraser was endorsed by the DFL caucus in the 1978 US Senate campaign but subsequently lost in the primaries to Bob Short, an anti–BWCAW Act candidate who gained support in the Arrowhead by framing Fraser as an urban elite environmentalist, uniformly opposed to the interests of working-class Iron Rangers.[58]

And the conflict continued. Truly, it has never stopped. In the early 1990s, a fight over a truck portage that transported boats between two lakes in the BWCAW led to years of litigation. A federal court finally ruled that the portage must be closed and that trucks were not allowed.[59] In recent years, the debates have included the placement of cellphone towers near (or potentially inside) the BWCAW and the permitting process for BWCAW visitors.[60]

Copper-nickel mining is now the latest but unlikely to be the last source of conflict over how to use the land and who gets to determine the future of northeastern Minnesota. Some of the same groups and people who were on opposing sides of the wilderness debates are still involved in the fight over copper-nickel mining. In my interviews and observations, I heard mining opponents and proponents alike raise issues from the 1950s and 1970s, even pointing out that they had not forgotten which families in Ely took which sides in the BWCAW fights. One summer evening while I was paddling on Burnside Lake nearly Ely, a middle-aged couple sitting on their dock struck up a conversation with me—in Ely, people bump into each other not only at the grocery store but also at boat launches and out on the lake. When I told the couple I was studying copper-nickel mining, they described the tensions in town, claiming these were "ancestral" conflicts with divisions steeped in longstanding family feuds over the BWCAW.

Iron Rangers' lamentations about federal overreach suggest still-gaping wounds: Tom, a retired miner, spoke bitterly about a family property lost to the Feds in the 1950s because it was located within the new BCWAW's boundaries, even as he drove me to his family's lakeside cabin outside Ely in 2017. Others pointed to restrictions on planes and motorboats, telling me the government had harmed the region's economy by cutting off revenue from the wealthy tourists who once came "up north" for extravagant fishing trips at fly-in resorts. Now, they would say, shaking their heads, environmentalists and government regulators wanted to stop copper-nickel-mining development—just another instance of outsiders hurting their community and disrespecting their way of life.

Environmental groups—especially those focused on the Twin Metals project, which is within the watershed of the BWCAW—for their part, frame the fight over copper-nickel mining as part of the ongoing effort to protect precious land and a dwindling wilderness experience. They see it as imperative to ensure that neither big industry nor small-town residents are left to determine how this place is used. The prospect of a large mine near the BWCAW is an anathema, an undoing of hard-won conservation protections and the end of pristine waters and quiet, dark nights. The new generation of conservationists is unwilling to make the sorts of compromises that have allowed carve-outs for mining in the watershed.

Fights over canoes and motorboats are, in some ways, proxy fights. They are also about different ways of understanding and experiencing nature, deeply linked to people's identities and sense of place (more on this in chapter 3).[61] Many supporters of motorized vehicles tend to be from rural northeastern Minnesota and identify as working class. For them, motorboats are part of how they relate to the place and the land, and restrictions symbolize the judgment of outsiders. Ardent wilderness supporters tend to come from urban and suburban areas across Minnesota and the US and have different social and class backgrounds. They see canoeing as a way to enjoy the pristine and quiet wilderness and see motorboats as a disruption to this cherished landscape.

Taking a step back, we can also recognize that land-use disputes between predominantly white settlers completely overlook thousands of years of Ojibwe and other Anishinaabe peoples' uninterrupted use of the same lands.[62] The historian Brenda Child, a member of the Red Lake Band of Chippewa (Ojibwe) Indians, describes a third perspective on the impact of Great Lakes conservation efforts: "From an Ojibwe perspective, the creation of national parks and forests within our homeland was part of a broader colonial history of appropriating Indigenous lands and resources."[63] Creating a wilderness area based on the imaginary of a pristine place untouched by humans necessarily involves the erasure of Indigenous history.[64] It can also create tensions between groups we might expect to align over conservation, because Indigenous people and tribes often prioritize exercising their treaty rights in wilderness areas, retaining the ability to maintain livelihoods and cultural practices through using the land.[65] That can result in settler conservationists interpreting Indigenous people's long-standing activities as disruptions to the untrammeled wilderness and barriers to *scientific* resource management.

The BWCAW is within the 1854 Treaty-ceded territory, and Ojibwe tribes do have rights to hunt, fish, and harvest in the area (currently, without needing to acquire entry permits like non-Native visitors), provided they follow BWCAW regulations with regard to motor vehicles and the collection of natural resources. Tribes argue that certain of these restrictions, such as not being able to use motorboats to harvest wild rice, infringe on their treaty rights. In the late 1990s, four members of the Bois Forte Band of Chippewa (Ojibwe) were arrested for violating this stricture. In court, they argued that tribes, not the US government, have the sole authority to regulate the actions of tribal members on treaty lands. They lost: in the landmark *US v. Gotchnik* case, a federal district judge ruled that the US government could regulate activities in a wilderness area and that nineteenth-century treaties did not enshrine Indigenous use of motorboats and ATVs.[66] The ruling did, however, affirm that tribal members could use motorized tools, such as electric drills for ice fishing, within the treaty lands and that creation of the BWCAW did not abrogate other treaty rights.

Indigenous groups have *also* clashed with pro-industry forces, which have proven even more hostile to tribal interests and treaty rights. Multiple-use proponents and extractive industries have resisted Indigenous use and control of land, particularly when tribes get in the way of industrial development and the unfettered recreation access of white, non-Native people. Groups of white hunters and anglers have even contested what they characterize as "special treatment"—the treaty concessions that allow for continued tribal use of wilderness areas and harvesting of plants and animals—on the grounds that everyone should be subject to the same regulations.[67] From the mid-1980s through the early 1990s, Ojibwe members exercising tribal fishing rights across Minnesota and Wisconsin were subject to violent backlash from white anglers in a conflict dubbed "The Walleye War."[68]

So, what happens when proud, working-class, rural residents; profit-seeking multinational mining corporations; Indigenous peoples; and conservationists and environmentalists collide in Minnesota's Arrowhead over copper-nickel-mining proposals? Let us find out.

2

Acceptance and Resistance

The Fight over Copper-Nickel Mining

In a city of just eighty-five thousand, it is notable for nearly a thousand people to show up for a government meeting. But on a blustery and cold Thursday afternoon in March 2017, the drab Duluth Entertainment Convention Center was packed for a US Forest Service public comment session. The lobby thronged with people pressing competing stickers and signs into the hands of citizens pouring out of coach buses—"We Support Mining," some said, and others, "Save the Boundary Waters." Here on the North Shore of Lake Superior, the US Forest Service was charged with studying the potential environmental impacts of withdrawing federal mineral leases in the Rainy River Watershed, which feeds into the BWCAW—including the leases needed for the proposed Twin Metals project.

With forty-five minutes until the hearing began, I walked down a stairwell, where my attention was drawn toward an overflowing conference room. I wedged myself in, finding a spot to stand in the very back of the room among the audience clad in jeans, hoodies adorned with union logos, and work boots, and listened to the press conference under way. A parade of copper-nickel-mining supporters, local politicians, union leaders, and industry representatives took the stage. When a white male in his fifties boomed into the mic that the Iron Range was "standing up" and was "here to fight," the crowd of mostly white, mostly middle-aged folks in pro-mining shirts, stickers, and hats hooted with approval. As the press conference ended, I slipped back outside the convention center, where a cadre of environmental organizations had just wrapped up their own press conference. Here, too, a crowd of mostly white people (albeit representing a larger age range, roughly early twenties through seventies) wearing puffy down jackets and hiking boots was preparing to march into the convention center together behind a "Save the Boundary Waters" banner.

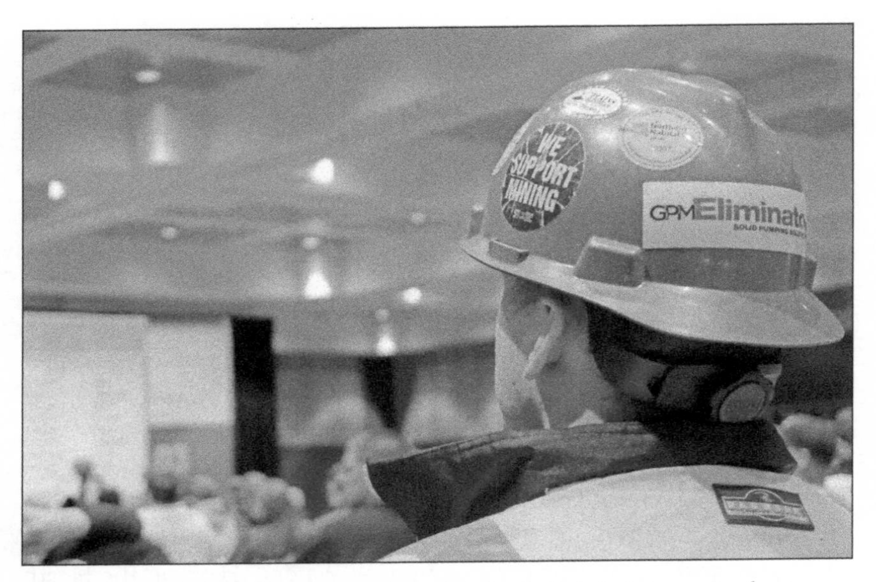

Pro-mining worker at a federal government hearing in Duluth, Minnesota, about copper-nickel mining in March 2017. (Photo by Erik Kojola)

By early 2017, copper-nickel mining was, as one journalist reported, "one of the most controversial environmental projects ever proposed in Minnesota."[1] Hearings like the session I described were setting records for public attendance and comments, and the issue was regularly in the news, even attracting national media coverage from publications like the *New York Times* and the *Washington Post* and political attention from US senators and representatives from Minnesota and other states. National environmental organizations and outdoor recreation and apparel companies like Patagonia and REI had begun to mobilize in support of local and statewide environmental groups critical of mining. Conservative Republicans from the Congressional Western Caucus descended on the Iron Range to show their support for copper-nickel mining, environmental deregulation, and industrial development and resource extraction on public lands.

To outsiders, this might all seem a bit odd. The region is proudly called the Iron Range. Iron mines have operated here for more than a century without much fuss, yet proposals about adding copper-nickel mines in a rural mining region proved incredibly controversial. Geography is part of the answer: extracting rich ore deposits has attracted a lot of capital and shaped the region's economy and culture. Towns were built—and then relocated—around iron mines. However, that same geology creates unique challenges and environmental risks. The landscape of boreal forests and hundreds of interconnected lakes where you can spend weeks, even months, paddling across a vast protected wilderness area adds contention, as people want to protect a cherished recreation place from industrial development. The prospect of noisy trucks, and round-the-clock explosions, along with the risk of water pollution to an area where you can still safely drink water straight out of a lake, is seen by some people as a threat and out of character with the place.

Taken together, the backdrop for copper-nickel-mining conflicts in Minnesota looks a lot like the context of fights over resource extraction throughout the country, from mountaintop removal coal mining in Appalachia to oil and gas fracking in Pennsylvania and New York to gold mining in Alaska. The prospect of new resource extraction brings promises of jobs and economic development to areas struggling with disinvestment. Yet the promised prosperity from extractive development rarely arrives. Instead, mining often creates booms and busts that leave behind poverty and environmental problems.[2] Industrial development risks ecosystems and public health and threatens other industries, including tourism and farming, that depend on a clean environment. Mining is often sited on or near Indigenous peoples' lands, imperiling their livelihoods, access to vital resources, and important cultural and spiritual sites, often violating tribal sovereignty and treaty rights.[3]

In this chapter, I provide an overview of current economic and social conditions in the Iron Range and describe the key differences between proposed copper-nickel mines and legacy iron mines. Then I detail PolyMet's NorthMet and Twin Metals' Minnesota projects, examining how and why the projects have become controversial and describing key turning points in their political advances.

A Snapshot of the Iron Range Today

Like so many of the country's other resource-extraction and industrial regions that have been battered by the uncertainties of boom-and-bust economies, communities in the Iron Range are feeling the effects of disinvestment and economic decline.[4] There are places where it is worse—Appalachia had a poverty rate near 20 percent in 2014, when it was just 13.5 percent in the Iron Range—but the past fifty years have not been kind.[5] Shifts in the global steel industry and mechanization of mining production have reduced the workforce needed to extract the same amount of iron ore.[6] A dearth of good-paying jobs, increased unemployment, rising poverty, and decreasing state revenues to fund public services have combined, leaving the Iron Range with higher unemployment and a lower household median income than the rest of Minnesota.[7]

The Iron Range is still a mining powerhouse: in 2016, its mines had the capacity to extract forty million tons of iron ore each year, or about 75 percent of total annual US iron-ore production. At the industry's peak in 1979, it employed sixteen thousand workers on the Iron Range; today just about forty-five hundred workers staff six operating iron mines, and across the entire state, just under sixty-five hundred people work in mining and logging.[8] One saving grace may be that nearly all of Minnesota's iron mines remain unionized, unlike mining operations in Appalachia, where coal companies busted unions, or in Western states, where few were ever unionized. Thus, the dwindling mining jobs are coveted—unionized, with decent benefits, retirement, and pay as high as $80,000–$90,000 a year.[9] The 2019 median hourly wage for mining-industry jobs in Minnesota's Arrowhead region was $37.32, compared to the overall median wage of $19.20. Few other manual and industrial sectors exist that can offer compensation packages that rival the quality of unionized mining jobs. These coveted, higher-paid mining jobs are held primarily by white men. In 2019, 92 percent of mining-industry workers in the region were men, although women made up 50.4 percent of the region's workers overall.[10]

As mining came to account for a smaller and smaller portion of employment and revenue in the region, a concurrent shift toward a service economy has pushed more residents into health care, retail, and food-service jobs. In 2016, 20 percent of Iron Rangers were employed in the health-care industry.[11] Tourism and hospitality are also significant, accounting for the employment of over seventeen thousand people and $900 million in sales across northeastern Minnesota in 2016.[12] The region has popular fishing, hunting, boating, and camping destinations, attracting locals and visitors from metro areas (though Minnesotans announcing they are "going up north" for a weekend getaway often mean going to any popular lake area north of the Twin Cities, not necessarily to the Iron Range). However, jobs in the service, health, and tourism sectors tend to be lower paid and come with fewer benefits than mining jobs do.[13] Many of these lower-paid industries also predominantly employ women.

Economic struggles contribute to a shrinking and aging population in the Iron Range. The population has slowly decreased over the past ninety years, a drain that began in the 1930s, when labor-intensive natural, high-grade iron mining reached its peak. Even the development of new taconite iron mines to extract and process low-grade ore in the 1950s and 1960s could not revive employment and population levels, because the process was getting so much less labor intensive. In Lake, St. Louis, and Itasca Counties (which make up the Iron Range), the population declined at least 30 percent from 1960 to 2014.[14] A second wave of depopulation crested when an iron-industry bust in the mid-2010s led to mine closures and slowdowns. Politicians, losing constituents, jobs, and the taxes that go with them, sounded the alarm.

With young people leaving to seek higher education and jobs elsewhere, the remaining population is "graying."[15] In 2016, more than a fifth of Iron Rangers were over age sixty-five (it was 15 percent in the rest of the state).[16] Fewer young people means fewer families having and raising children. The smaller, older population has severely constricted the enrollment and funding in Iron Range schools, which were once a source of community pride. Hibbing's high school building, with an ornate two-story Jacobean Revival façade, an indoor pool (the first US high school to have one), and an eighteen-hundred-seat auditorium modeled on the Capitol Theatre in New York and decorated with Belgian chandeliers adorned in Czech crystal, cost an impressive $4 million to construct in 1940. The building, known as the "castle in the woods," was lauded by the national press for its grandeur and offered evidence that mining revenue could be channeled toward improving the community.[17] Those auditorium seats are rarely filled these days, as student enrollment dropped by half between 1998 and 2015. The ornate building needs upkeep and repairs that local governments cannot fund.[18] Throughout my interviews, Iron Range residents and leaders counted high-quality schools among the region's assets while worrying over their future. In Ely, a woman in her late fifties asked plaintively, "What do you do when your high school goes from graduating classes of 150 to 200 students, down to 37 this year? What does that tell you about a town? It's saying it's not sustainable, that the way things are now, the town cannot sustain itself."

The remaining, aging populace has different needs and preferences than younger generations do. I met people in their twenties and thirties, even forties, who felt like it was the "old-timers" who were adamantly pro-mining. The younger generation did not experience the heyday of mining and do not have the same economic and cultural ties to mining. This is not to say that younger Iron Rangers are anti-mining but rather that they are more ambivalent and not waiting for copper-nickel mining to rescue the economy. On a summer afternoon, I went into one of the small liquor stores in Ely to buy a six-pack of beer, and when the young male clerk found out I was studying copper-nickel mining, he lamented that many old-timers saw new mining as a savior. He thought copper-nickel mining would not solve the region's economic woes, which required more diversification and creation of new industries.

A New and Different Type of Mining

Understanding why copper-nickel-mining development is controversial requires looking at the differences between these nonferrous metals and iron (*the* ferrous metal), particularly the additional environmental risks raised by this new type of mining, the different economic drivers of the copper and nickel industries, and the different locations of proposed copper-nickel mines.[19]

Copper is the most abundant metal in the Duluth Complex deposit in northeastern Minnesota. It is the key material that corporations hope to extract, alongside nickel, gold, palladium, silver, cobalt, chromium, and zinc. While copper has been used by humans for centuries, it became crucial for industrial society since it is an excellent electrical conductor; copper makes up the electrical wires that keep factories running, light up cities, and power computers.[20] The metal's ubiquity in modern society—embedded in almost every consumer and industrial good from buildings to cars to cellphones—has made it a sort of economic bellwether.[21] In ten years alone, 2005 to 2015, global consumption rose 38 percent, and analysts predict steady demand for copper well into the future.[22] Industry boosters like to point out that copper, as well as nickel, is essential for creating a sustainable economy and renewable energy since it is used in things like solar panels and batteries—both a challenge for supplying the material needs of energy transitions and a way to paint a green veneer over what is usually seen as a dirty, grey industry.

A mining project's profit forecast depends, in large part, on the price of metals to be sold on global markets. Corporate decisions to finance and build new mining projects in Minnesota rest on the prices of copper and other metals, but these are shaped by the complex processes of global demand, financialization, and speculation. According to industry analysts, copper is highly sought, yet it is a risky sector: its prices oscillate quickly in reaction to broader global market conditions, like increases or decreases in Chinese construction and consumption.[23] Markets for copper and other natural resource commodities have also become increasingly financialized in the past forty years. Speculative financial tools such as futures and derivatives trading help separate the price of a commodity from the underlying use of the physical asset—prices do not follow simple supply and demand trends.[24] For natural resources markets, this can mean increasing price volatility and amplifying booms and busts.[25] A period of global economic growth, particularly in Global South countries, saw a spike in copper and other metal prices in the early 2000s.[26] Mining-industry revenues hit record highs in 2007.[27] This is when PolyMet and Twin Metals were developing plans to mine what appeared to be financially attractive, low-grade deposits in Minnesota. The Great Recession put an abrupt end to that, disrupting financial markets, bottoming out US housing construction, and slowing China's economic expansion; then prices rebounded.[28] Though currently the price of copper appears steady in the short term, it is volatile and creates uncertainty, which puts pressures on mining companies to reduce their operating costs, including limiting spending on labor and environmental protections.

Globalization in the mining industry has also changed the pressures, logics, and strategies driving the actions of corporations developing new copper-nickel mines. The mining industry is dominated by large multinational corporations (MNCs), which invest in, construct, and operate mines around the world. MNCs are becoming broader industrial, commodity, and financial companies that generate profits through speculation, finance, and trading. Glencore, which owns a majority stake in PolyMet, is one of the world's largest commodity-trading companies, with a network of more than eighty subsidiaries and 150 mines, shipping terminals, refineries, and warehouses around the world, and over $200 billion in annual revenue.[29] Small, "junior" mining companies, including PolyMet and Twin Metals, often conduct initial prospecting, exploration, and permitting, with the goal of attracting investors and being purchased by the MNCs, which have the capital to build and operate large industrial mining facilities.[30] Large corporations are able to avoid the initial risks of exploration while enjoying profits producing and selling metals.

A final complexity is introduced by the shifting international investment relations as firms from the Global South—in a reversal of historical trends—are developing extractive projects in the Global North.[31] For example, Chilean mining firms like Antofagasta, which owns Twin Metals, are now formidable, financing projects around the world.[32] Meanwhile, Glencore's operations are largely in the Global South, so PolyMet would be its first US operation; some observers believe that the PolyMet mine is a strategy for Glencore to expand into less risky locations as the company withstands criticism over its human rights and environmental practices in the Global South.[33]

Environmental Impacts of Copper-Nickel Mining

Copper mines dating back to the Roman Empire have polluted surrounding waterways, and some of these ancient mines continue to produce toxic water.[34] In contemporary history, copper and other nonferrous (also called "hardrock") mines are major sources of water pollution, air pollution, and occupational and public health hazards. Hardrock mining is one of the largest sources of US Environmental Protection Agency (EPA) Superfund sites.[35] One of the largest and most iconic is in Butte, Montana, where a shuttered copper mine has flooded to form the Berkeley Pit, which has become a tourist destination for people seeking to experience the awe of large-scale industrial pollution.[36] Mining creates a host of environmental injustices around the world, as the industry exposes nearby communities to pollution and damages workers' health through toxic chemicals and physical injury in a workplace that is notorious for being dangerous and dirty.[37]

In Minnesota, copper-nickel mining is environmentally riskier than existing iron mining is. This is due to the location of the new mines and the different geochemistry of the ore. Copper, nickel, and other nonferrous metals are often found in rocks bonded to sulfide minerals, which produce sulfuric acid when they are exposed to air and water—what regulators and industry officials call "acid mine drainage."[38] In contrast, Minnesota's iron ore typically has fewer sulfide minerals and contains other minerals that can buffer acid generation.[39] The copper and nickel deposits in the Duluth Complex are also low grade, ranging from 0.25 percent to 0.66 percent copper, which means generating enormous amounts of waste in order to access a small share of valuable metals.[40] As much as 97 percent of extracted ore will be leftover tailings—the nonvaluable waste rock.[41] And it is this waste rock that can create acid mine drainage, which contaminates drinking water, damages aquatic ecosystems, and kills aquatic plants and animals. Acidic water also leaches heavy metals out of the surrounding rocks, many of which are identified by the World Health Organization as major public health concerns, such as arsenic, cadmium, lead, and mercury.[42] Mercury alone is a neurotoxin that bioaccumulates in fish, causing health problems when consumed by humans and disproportionately impacting pregnant women and children.[43] The potential that tailings will create acid mine drainage is pernicious, continuing into perpetuity because the sulfides cannot be removed, nor can the chemical process creating sulfuric acid be reversed.

There is extensive evidence showing that copper-nickel mining in the Iron Range has the potential to create acid mine drainage, though the precise amount of sulfides and extent of acid mine drainage is contested.[44] Deposits have different amounts of sulfides; thus, ore from the NorthMet mine may generate different amounts of acid than at the Twin Metals site.[45] Further, different landscapes have varying "buffering capacity"—waterbodies can potentially mitigate the effects of acid mine drainage by lowering pH levels. Some scientists, state agencies, and industry representatives claim that environmentalists exaggerate the threat of acid mine drainage. They insist that the Duluth Complex ores have a relatively low potential to generate acids compared to ores mined in other places.[46]

Sulfates from mining runoff is a particular concern in Minnesota because sulfates damage wild rice (*manoomin* in Ojibwe, meaning "the good fruit" or "spirit delicacy," and *Psiŋ* in Dakota), a unique grain that grows in ecosystems of the Great Lakes region. Wild rice is culturally, spiritually, nutritionally, and economically vital for Anishinaabe and Dakota peoples.[47] Wild rice was a quick favorite among the region's white settlers, and today it is part of the state's identity (earning it the honor of being Minnesota's state grain). In 1973, the state legislature, aiming to protect wild rice, implemented the country's only regulatory standard on sulfate emission levels: ten milligrams per liter.[48] Runoff from the copper-nickel mines is expected to break the barrier, raising alarm among those who note that wild rice has deteriorated precipitously since colonization and industrialization of the area.[49]

Sulfates also accelerate mercury methylation, the process of turning mercury into methyl mercury, the form that is toxic to humans.[50] As I mentioned briefly, methyl mercury is already a public health concern in this area of northern Minnesota. Many lakes and rivers have unsafe mercury levels, and public health warnings suggest limiting consumption of some wild-caught fish species, especially by pregnant women.[51] Thus, any leakage from copper-nickel mining would be on top of the already elevated levels, compounding risks to women, children, and Indigenous people.[52]

The standard approach to storing tailings is to dump them into a basin created by walls of soil and rock that serve as a dam to hold thousands of gallons of water and sludge. This pond is then covered with water, soil, or synthetic materials, all intended but by no means guaranteed to protect against water containing toxins and acidic water from spilling, seeping, and leeching its way into Iron Range water and soil. These structures are expected to operate for hundreds, even thousands, of years, but there are often leaks. The walls are prone to erosion, weakening, and shifting. It is rare, but tailings dams have collapsed. And there is some evidence that failure rates have actually accelerated in the past thirty years, despite advancements in technology and engineering.[53] Environmental groups cite the 2005 Mount Polley disaster in Canada as a cautionary tale: when a tailings basin collapsed at an operating copper mine, causing a massive spill of twenty-four million cubic meters of mine waste that flooded downstream waters and destroyed surrounding forests.[54] A newer approach to storing this hazardous material is called "dry stacking," which is generally seen as the safer, more expensive option.[55] PolyMet proposed a tailings dam in its permit applications, while Twin Metals, under immense pressure, proposed dry-stack tailings storage in its preliminary plans.[56]

Mining companies have proposed technical solutions to treat wastewater and runoff, but the adequacy and financial feasibility is hotly debated. The building and operation of technology like reverse osmosis water treatment is expensive, and at this scale, its efficacy is uncertain.[57] Like tailings storage, water treatment and containment systems rarely work exactly according to plan. Mine engineers hired by Earthworks, an environmental organization, report that the actual amount of water pollution and acid mine drainage from hardrock mines in the US is frequently underestimated in environmental assessments and that mitigation efforts frequently fail.[58] Again, the threat of leeching heavy metals is one without end. Wastewater needs to be stored and treated for thousands of years.[59] Regulators and environmental advocates are concerned that the time horizon of potential pollution extends well beyond the life span of a water treatment system or a single company.[60] There is no real way to know whether the containment strategies will work in perpetuity.

The wet climate of northeastern Minnesota brings extra hazards, especially compared to the arid climates in which most other US copper mines are located. Heavy rainfall can overwhelm tailings basins and water treatment systems, leading to spills.[61] As climate change contributes to stronger, less predictable storms and weather events, these risks multiply.[62] In a vastly interconnected waterway landscape like northeastern Minnesota's, water pollution could spread rapidly, widely, and with nasty consequences.[63]

Other environmental issues arise from the impacts of large-scale land-use change and industrial activity that destroys wetlands, disrupts wildlife habitat, and generates noise, light, and air pollution. Extracting copper, nickel, and other metals is done by digging tunnels thousands of feet underground or removing the surface soil to expose the valuable veins of metal, thus creating large open pits. In both underground and surface mines, explosives are used to dislodge the ore, which is scooped up by large mechanical shovels and loaded into trucks or trains for transport to a processing facility, which can generate dust and requires large amounts of energy.[64]

Finally, we cannot overlook the potential for any new mines to create health risks for workers and nearby residents. Occupational health advocates argue that there are many uncertain risks with copper-nickel mining and that current safety regulations are scientifically outdated.[65] Dust released during the mining process and from transporting ore can harm human health because it contains amphibole fibers (which are similar to asbestos).[66] Physicians and public health professionals continue to raise concerns about the potential long-term public and occupational health impacts of both proposed projects.[67]

Minnesota's regulations for nonferrous mining differ from its regulations for iron mining.[68] The Minnesota Mineland Reclamation Act, passed in 1969, lays out rules for site reclamation; it was updated in 1993 with specific rules for nonferrous mining. The state has financial assurance laws applying to nonferrous mining that require companies to provide funds to pay for the costs of cleanup and reclamation when a mine is closed and if its owner does not perform the necessary cleanup. Environmental groups and some lawmakers are concerned that the financial assurance laws may be inadequate for accurately estimating future costs of cleaning up copper-nickel mining, mostly because Minnesota has never issued a permit for a nonferrous mine and so its regulatory system is untested.

Threats to Indigenous Livelihoods and Treaty Rights

Copper-nickel mining is a risk to Ojibwe people, whose livelihoods, health, and cultural practices including hunting, fishing, and gathering depend on having clean air, soil, and water. Tribes contend that the inevitable pollution and land-use changes accompanying the new mines would harm fisheries and damage habitat for deer, moose, and other animals. Of vital concern is the impact on wild rice (*manoomin*), an important food source for Minnesota's Indigenous people and a sacred plant that is seen as their relative and is prominent in Anishinaabe prophecies and origin stories.[69] Pollution would further risk the health of these already-overburdened communities, where, for example, increased mercury levels in aquatic ecosystems and fish will disproportionately impact Indigenous communities, for which fishing is both a cultural practice and a major food source.

Pollution that harms plants and nonhuman animals could violate the 1854 Treaty between the US government and the Fond du Lac, Boise Forte, and Grand Portage Bands of Lake Superior Chippewa (Ojibwe). The treaty granted tribal members the right to hunt, fish, and gather on and off reservation lands in what is now northeastern Minnesota. The proposed mines are on territory ceded in the treaty, and any pollution will inexorably impact lands and waters in the area.[70] US courts have upheld the treaty rights of tribal members across territories ceded in the 1854 and other treaties (these are called "usufructuary rights"). Yet treaty rights are meaningless if there are no fish, deer, or wild rice to be fished, hunted, and gathered due to water and air pollution, habitat loss, and land development. Tribes across the US have found some legal success, arguing in court that pollution that damages plant and wildlife habitat is a treaty violation, and they have been able to stop or alter a number of extractive development projects.[71] Treaty rights and Indigenous sovereignty are not the focus of this book, but numerous Indigenous and allied scholars and activists have written about these issues in Minnesota and across the US.[72] I do examine how, or if, white settlers talk about Indigenous people and treaty rights and how dominant discourses construct the land as open for development—a practice rife in the US's history of extractive settler colonialism.[73]

Constructing new mine sites adds another threat: it may disrupt Indigenous cultural, spiritual, and burial sites, which are protected under US and international law. Building large open-pit mines, processing facilities, and heavy-haul roads would transform the land that Anishinaabe and Dakota people have lived on for millennia, and it would destroy important spiritual and cultural places. Under the National Environmental Policy Act (NEPA) and National Historic Preservation Act, government agencies are instructed to assess impacts to American Indian religious, historical, and cultural sites before moving forward with such projects. However, as with many promises made by the US government to tribal nations, these assessments are often limited and lack the power to actually stop a project.

Legacies of Contested Copper-Nickel Mining

The wave of proposals to develop copper-nickel mines in Minnesota that swelled in the early 2000s was not the first. An earlier boom in exploration and investment, in the 1960s and '70s, did not result in any actual construction, yet its history laid the groundwork for contemporary conflicts. These fifty-year-old fights demonstrate how environmental concerns, regulatory and political decisions, and global commodity prices all matter when it comes to determining whether industrial development happens.

The nonferrous-metal deposits in the Duluth Complex were first identified in 1948 by researchers and mining companies, which sparked commercial exploration and investments through the 1950s and '60s.[74] Amid a nascent environmental movement and worries about impact to the BWCAW, the public responded with concern. Then-governor Wendell Anderson created an interagency task force on copper-nickel mining in 1972 to study the issue and concluded that mining was feasible.[75] Within two years, a pair of companies—International Nickel Company and Amax—prepared applications to get mining projects approved for construction. Yet the state legislature put the projects on hold, commissioning a comprehensive assessment of social and environmental impacts. It took five years to complete *The Minnesota Regional Copper-Nickel Study*—the period was a sort of de facto moratorium on mining. When the report came out in 1979, the price of copper and nickel had dropped, and the low-grade ore deposit was deemed unprofitable.[76] Eventually, companies sold off their mineral leases and abandoned their plans.[77]

Copper-nickel mining largely dropped from public debate until global prices spiked again in the early 2000s, which brought new exploration and investment. At first, this was a low-profile issue about regulatory procedures and economic development. However, copper-nickel mining would grow into one of the most contested environmental issues in Minnesota history.

PolyMet's NorthMet Project: New Mining on Top of Old Mining

PolyMet's proposed NorthMet mine would cover thirty square miles and include a seven-hundred-foot-deep open-pit mine connected with

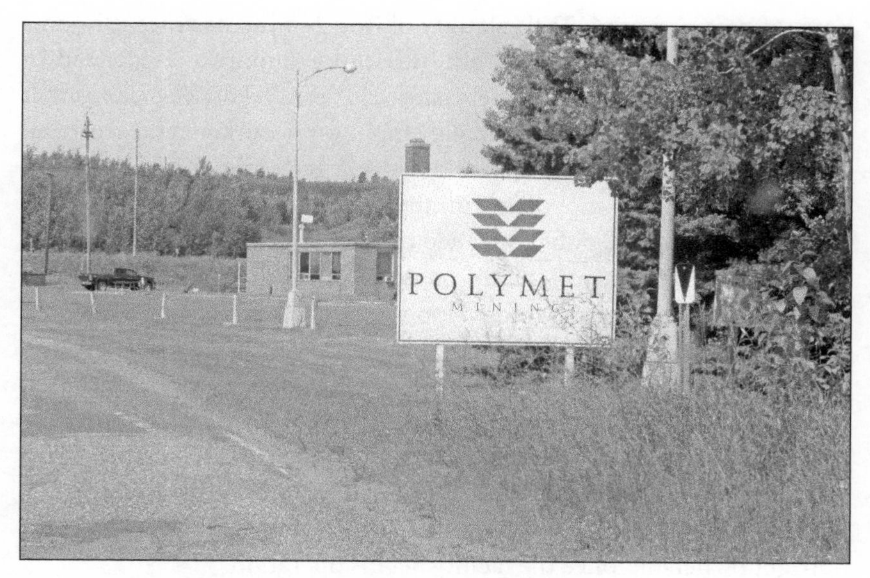

PolyMet proposes to repurpose an old iron-mining facility and create a new open-pit mine. (Photo by Erik Kojola)

a seven-mile train track to a processing plant.[78] The site is six miles south of Babbitt, Minnesota, and six miles north of Hoyt Lakes and Aurora, Minnesota—small towns built by iron-mining companies in the 1940s and '50s. The plan involves mining on previously undeveloped land, including 6,650 federal acres within the Superior National Forest. However, mining on national forest land is not allowed.[79] Thus, in order to access these potentially stranded assets, the company proposed a land swap: it would hand over 6,722 acres of private land in other parts of northern Minnesota in exchange for the federal land above the ore deposit.[80] Constructing the mine would destroy sixteen thousand acres of wetlands, meaning it would be the largest single permitted impact to wetlands in Minnesota history.[81] The company would also repurpose LTV Steel's old iron-ore processing facility and tailings basin.

The nearby small towns, like many up here, are struggling. LTV Steel in Hoyt Lakes closed in 2011, laying off fourteen hundred workers (many residents and local leaders are now hopeful that PolyMet may resurrect the facility). The Northshore Mine, just a mile from the proposed NorthMet site, is still in operation, though ups and downs forced closures for parts of 2015 and 2016. The volatility of iron mining has meant booms and busts for the towns' communities and economies, evidenced in school consolidations and grocery-store closures.[82] PolyMet claims that the $1 billion project will eventually employ 360 workers and create an additional 600 spin-off jobs, such as jobs in restaurants and retail and equipment suppliers supporting mining operations.

PolyMet is a small, publicly traded company—a "junior mining company," in industry terms—that is based in Canada. It has no other operations and was formed to develop the NorthMet project. However, some of the major global players in mining have invested in the project, namely, the Swiss-based Glencore.[83] By 2019, Glencore had purchased over three-quarters of PolyMet's stock, and it holds rights to purchase the initial minerals once operation begins.[84] Glencore has already provided the capital to fund operating costs, allowing PolyMet to move forward with the project and prompting speculation that Glencore will take outright ownership once the facility begins operation.[85]

PolyMet claims that the mine can operate without significant impacts to the surrounding ecosystem and waterways in the St. Louis River watershed (which flows through the city of Duluth before draining into Lake Superior).[86] It is an area that has already experienced a long history of industrialization, having played host to the bulk of the state's iron mining. The NorthMet project is also seventy miles upstream of the Fond du Lac Band of Lake Superior Chippewa (Ojibwe) reservation along the St. Louis River. The tribe, directly in the path of potential pollution, has described the project as an "existential threat" to its reservation, forty-two hundred tribal members, and other Ojibwe and Indigenous people in the region.[87] Water is fundamental to Ojibwe livelihoods and culture—the Ojibwe name of the Fond du Lac Reservation is, in fact, *Nagaajiwanaang*, meaning "where the water stops," in reference to the slowing current of the St. Louis River before it enters Lake Superior.[88] The mine could damage some of the best wildlife and wild rice habitat in the region, destroy ecologically important peat lands, and result in the loss of lands in the 1854 Treaty territory.[89]

The Fond du Lac and Grand Portage Bands (the latter located farther north up the shore of Lake Superior) are also concerned about impacts to religious and historical sites and have critiqued the assessment of damage to cultural resources by government agencies as wholly inadequate.[90] Some potential impacts include damage to parts of the Laurentian Divide (*Mesabe Widjiu* in Ojibwe), a spiritually as well as geologically important place, and historic trails used by Indigenous people to travel, trade, and hunt.[91] Government agencies have largely declined to engage substantively with these complaints. As part of the environmental review process, PolyMet commissioned a study on the impact to tribal cultural resources and spiritual sites. The study, which involved interviews with elders and archeological surveys, was as fraught and limited as scholars might anticipate. In part, this is because traditional Indigenous knowledge is not legible to Western government institutions, which demand evidence and proof in the form of quantifiable metrics. It would be hard not to read a bit of a sneer into an environmental review document describing tribes' knowledge about their own cultural sites and history as lacking "specificity and verifiability."[92]

The NorthMet project began as routine mining exploration and received little public attention. In 1998, PolyMet bought mineral leases in the area and started exploratory studies. By 2004, the company had submitted preliminary mine plans to state agencies, triggering an environmental impact statement (EIS).[93] An EIS evaluates environmental and socioeconomic impacts but does not determine whether a project should be approved—the report is only a source of information meant to guide permitting decisions. PolyMet anticipated moving quickly through the EIS process and predicted that permits would be issued by 2006 and production could begin by 2007.[94] Those optimistic projections proved gravely mistaken. As of 2022, the project is still entangled in permitting and litigation. No construction has begun.

When the project was first proposed, environmental groups and Ojibwe tribes expressed their concerns about potential pollution and ecological disruptions, but public attention was limited. Newspaper coverage was scarce and only occasionally mentioned the environmental hazards of the project.[95] Things changed when, in 2010, the US EPA took the unusual action of deeming PolyMet's initial draft EIS inadequate and "environmentally unsatisfactory."[96] A lawyer with an environmental organization told me that this was an extremely rare action—only 3 percent of EISs receive an unsatisfactory rating.[97] This move meant a regulatory delay and an influx of public attention, as it seemed to legitimate environmentalists' and tribes' critiques of the proposal.[98] PolyMet had to create a supplemental EIS to address questions raised by the EPA, including about the adequacy of water-pollution modeling and risks from acid mine drainage.

The supplemental EIS process brought even more scrutiny and regulatory oversight. The US Forest Service and the Minnesota Department of Natural Resources (MNDNR) joined the Army Corps as co-lead agencies in conducting the revised environmental review—indicating their level of concern—and the company hired more staff, including a former commissioner of the Minnesota Pollution Control Agency.[99] The Bois Forte, Grand Portage, and Fond du Lac Bands, along with the 1854 Treaty Authority, an organization that manages natural resources within the treaty territory, and the Great Lakes Indian Fish and Wildlife Commission (GLIFWC), an organization that coordinates eleven tribes with treaty rights across the Upper Midwest, joined as cooperating agencies, too. Early drafts went to these groups for review, and the tribes were consulted through a semiformal but nonbinding process in which they had no decision-making authority.

By the early 2010s, opposition to PolyMet was strong.[100] Coverage in the state's two major newspapers, the *Star Tribune* and the *Duluth News-Tribune*, spiked around the 2010 EPA decision, then again during the 2013 and 2014 public comment periods and state elections in which the PolyMet mine was an important issue. Over thirty-five hundred people submitted public comments on the NorthMet EIS draft in 2010—the comments dwarfed the usual several hundred and were described by one reporter as "mini tidal wave."[101] Sensing some momentum, environmental groups expanded their public-awareness efforts. The groups stopped short of calls to block the mine, instead asking for rigorous environmental review and expanded pollution controls and financial assurances. The state's major mainstream environmental groups—the Minnesota Center for Environmental Advocacy (MCEA), the Sierra Club Northstar Chapter, the Izaak Walton League, and Conservation Minnesota—were active on the issue, as were smaller and locally focused groups such as the Friends of the Boundary Waters and WaterLegacy. MCEA, Conservation Minnesota, and Friends of the Boundary Waters formed a coalition called Mining Truth in May 2012 to focus on raising public awareness about the perils of copper-nickel mining.[102] Mining critics even took to the streets, such as a 2011 protest rally outside a PolyMet officials' meeting at the Minnesota Chamber of Commerce office in Duluth.[103]

This more visible opposition contributed to a countermobilization by mining supporters, including Iron Range politicians, business and industry groups, and construction and mining unions. Support for copper-nickel mining grew from the public-relations efforts of a few mining companies to a pro-mining social mobilization and public-relations campaign. In 2012, the Minnesota Building and Construction Trades Council and the Minnesota Chamber of Commerce formed the Jobs for Minnesotans coalition to promote development projects including oil and gas pipelines and copper-nickel mining.[104] Soon, the coalition expanded to include other companies and industry groups, local unions, cities, and community groups. Today, the organization has a small staff and operating budget focused on creating public-relations materials, hosting events, and commenting on legislation and regulatory decisions.

When the supplementary draft EIS was released to the public in January 2014, the comment period was twice as long as legally required (ninety rather than forty-five days) to account for the high amount of public concern.[105] There were a record-setting fifty-two thousand comments—ten times the previous state record for public comments on an EIS and nearly fifteen times as many comments as were submitted on the first EIS in 2010.[106] Three packed public comment sessions were held in St. Paul and towns in northern Minnesota. State and federal agencies had to develop new procedures to accommodate this influx of input. In November 2015, the preliminary final EIS, clocking in at a hefty thirty-five hundred pages, was released to the public, with more hearings held and record-setting numbers of public comments submitted—nearly sixty thousand this time.[107]

Mine critics were successful in generating public awareness. Minnesotans' support for the PolyMet project, measured in 2014 *Star Tribune* polls, decreased from 46 percent in February to 40 percent in September.[108] Polls by the Minnesota Environmental Partnership demonstrated public understanding of and opposition to copper-nickel mining, such that project support fell from 66 percent in 2009 to 35 percent in 2017 and project opposition rose from 19 percent to 52 percent. That same poll found more people reporting being aware of the issue; survey respondents with no opinion on the issue dropped from 22 percent to 9 percent.[109]

Surrounded by mounting critiques from environmental groups, public health professionals, tribes, and a critical public, the federal agencies nonetheless approved PolyMet's final EIS in March 2016. This was no rubber stamp for the project. PolyMet could only then begin the process of applying for over twenty state and federal permits. This meant another series of public hearings and comment sessions. Despite opposition, the NorthMet project eventually secured several key permit approvals from state and federal agencies. The MNDNR approved the Permit to Mine, the largest and most complicated permit and the first ever issued for nonferrous mining in Minnesota. Air and water permits were approved by the Minnesota Pollution Control Agency (MPCA). And in another major milestone, the USFS approved the land-swap proposal, in which PolyMet would trade the agency 6,690 acres of private land scattered across northern Minnesota for 6,650 acres of lands in the Superior National Forest. All of these actions were quickly met with lawsuits by environmental organizations; and as of early 2022, many are still in various stages of litigation, and approval remains in limbo. State and federal court decisions have been mixed, with some supporting environmentalists' arguments and others moving the project forward, siding with PolyMet.

Regardless of what politicians and courts decide, the fate of the project may come down to global finances and markets. A lingering issue is the amount of financial assurance PolyMet is required to provide for the costs of environmental cleanup in case of accident or bankruptcy. Critics and outside analysists doubt that PolyMet, a junior mining company with few assets, can actually secure the necessary financial backing.[110] Industry supporters and opponents alike concede that the global price of copper and nickel remains a deciding factor in whether the mine is constructed—much as it was in the 1970s. The estimated costs of the NorthMet project continue rising; in 2018, PolyMet estimated a cost of $1 billion, up from $650 million in 2015, which has added pressure on the company to attract investment, generate high revenues, and keep labor and environmental protection costs low.[111] Opponents find some hope in the project's financial precarity and believe further delays could lead investors to pull out and Glencore to lose interest in financing a project that looks less profitable.

Twin Metals' Minnesota Project: Mining on the Edge of the BWCAW

Twin Metals plans to extract copper, nickel, gold, and other metals through an underground mine located nine miles from Ely and just five miles from the edge of the BWCAW, near the South Kawishiwi River and Birch Lake—all of which is in the Rainy River watershed that feeds into the BWCAW. A prefeasibility document from 2014 showed plans for a $2.8 billion underground mine at depths up to forty-five hundred feet using over twenty-seven thousand acres of mineral leases that could process twenty thousand tons of ore per day—larger in both area and volume than PolyMet's project.[112] Twin Metals estimates that its mine would operate for twenty-five years, directly employ seven hundred people, and create fifteen hundred spin-off jobs during its operation.[113] However, after decisions by the Biden administration in 2021 to rescind the company's mineral leases, the project appears to be canceled, but Twin Metals is challenging those actions in court.

Yet again, global capital is interested in what lies below the soils of northeastern Minnesota. Twin Metals, like PolyMet, is a junior mining company, but it is a subsidiary of Chilean Antofagasta PLC, one of the world's largest producers of copper.[114] Antofagasta has played an important role in providing funding and political support for Twin Metals. For example, in 2010, chairman Jean-Paul Luksic, the son of Chilean billionaire Andronico Luksic, joined the Chilean ambassador to the US in a meeting with Minnesota's then-governor Tim Pawlenty and state legislators to discuss the project, which would be Antofagasta's first in the US.[115]

Water pollution is a major concern because waters in the BWCAW are largely unpolluted, and parts of the nearby Kawishiwi River are designated as "outstanding resource waters" (the highest level of water quality). Any pollution here would have significant impacts and is subject to strict standards.[116] The lakes and rivers in the BWCAW have low acidity and a low buffering capacity. Thus, BWCAW waters are at a heightened risk for mine-related degradation and acid mine drainage.[117] In response, Twin Metals has proposed various plans to prevent and mitigate pollution and potential water contamination. The company claims that the mine would produce no acid mine drainage because the ore has low sulfide content and tailings will be stored in dry stacks, avoiding the risk of dam failure and spills associated with the storage methods in the PolyMet proposal.[118]

Twin Metals is proposing an underground mine, but there are still impacts on the surface from construction, storing equipment, and transporting materials. This would occur on US Forest Service land that has never been mined and is part of a large expanse of undeveloped boreal forest; this unique ecosystem is an important habitat for wildlife including lynx, wolves, and moose and features some of the darkest skies and best stargazing in North America.[119] Noise from trucks and construction equipment, vibrations from explosions, and light from facilities could disrupt animals and plants and impact the wilderness experience.[120]

Opposition and Wilderness Conservation

Development of Twin Metals' Minnesota project began after PolyMet's project and entered the regulatory process in the midst of controversy. Thus, Twin Metals quickly gained state and national political attention and media coverage, including in outlets such as the *New York Times*, the *Washington Post*, the *Progressive*, *National Geographic*, and *Sierra* (the national newsletter of the Sierra Club). At the local level, debates over this project have roiled the town of Ely, where the dual histories of the region's resource extraction and outdoor recreation converge.[121] Ely was one of the earliest mining towns in the Iron Range but is also known as "the gateway to the Boundary Waters"; the main street is dotted with canoe outfitters, guiding companies, coffee shops, and small hotels. Ely is dealing with many of the same challenges as other Iron Range towns: a shrinking and aging population, poverty, and unemployment. The town of Ely's population has declined by nearly half since its peak of around six thousand in the 1930s, and 21 percent of Ely residents are over age sixty-five, compared to 15 percent of the overall state population.[122] The town's economic struggles include a 15 percent poverty rate and a median household income just above half the state's average.[123]

One quickly sees these tensions when one visits Ely. Yards are sprinkled with competing "Save the Boundary Waters" and "Mining Supports

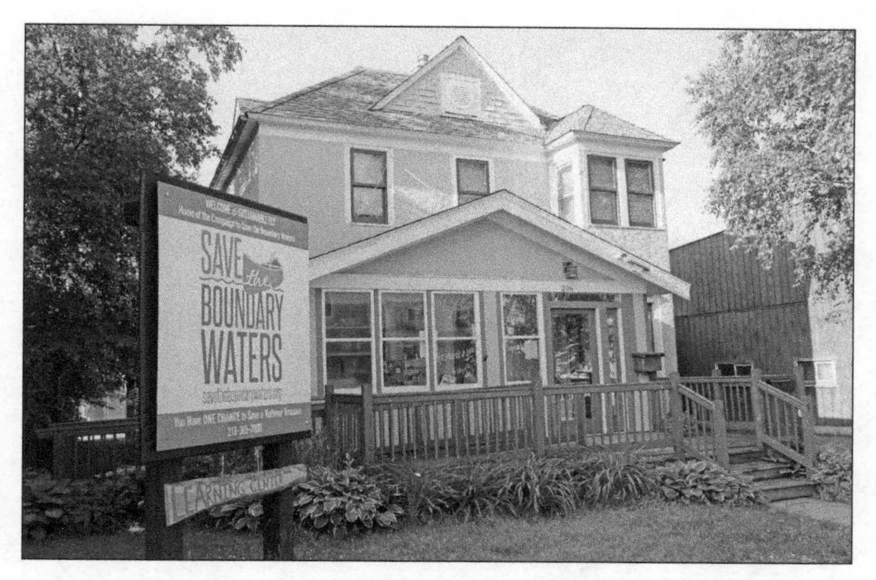

The Ely headquarters of Campaign to Save the Boundary Waters on East Sheridan Street in downtown. (Photo by Erik Kojola)

Us" signs, and the offices of the pro-mining group Up North Jobs and of the Campaign to Save the Boundary Waters, the leaders of mining opposition, sit a few blocks from each other on the main street through downtown. While I was checking into an aging motel on the edge of downtown during a winter fieldwork trip, the receptionist asked me what brought me to town—few tourists come in the dead of winter, and most of the rooms were vacant. When I told her that I was a researcher studying copper-nickel mining, she quickly remarked that the Twin Metals project was very controversial up here. She kept her cards close, not offering any hint of her views. Residents and community leaders in and around Ely are divided over hope that new mining will bring jobs and prosperity and fears the mining will bring pollution, damaging the tourism industry and repelling new residents.

While the population of Ely remains predominantly longtime residents, areas outside the town's boundaries have a growing population of summer vacationers, retirees, people working in tourism, and teleworkers who buy houses and cabins closer to lakes and the BWCAW.

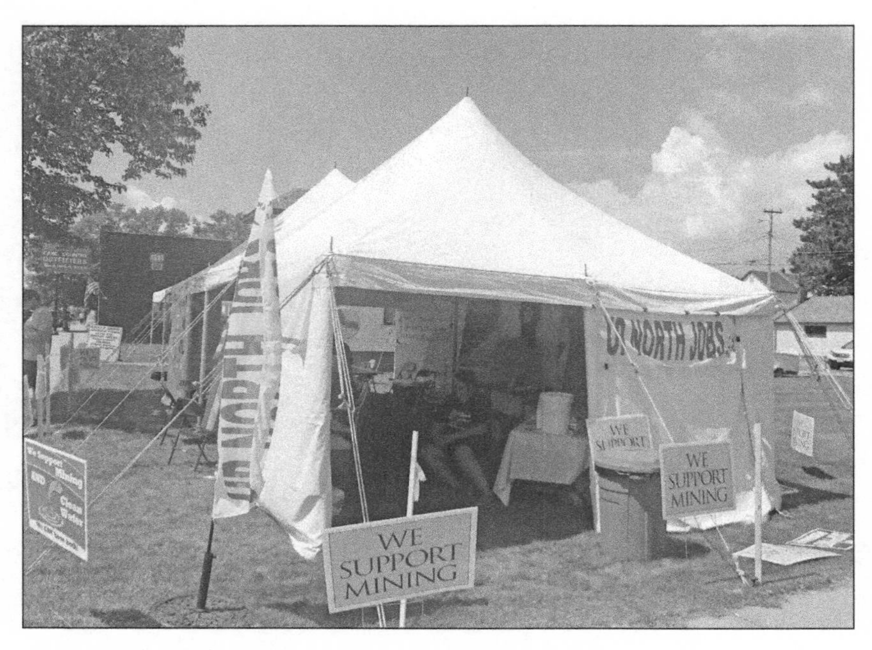

Pro-mining booth for a summer festival in Ely, Minnesota. (Photo by Erik Kojola)

As of 2015, the townships surrounding Ely had a larger percentage of adults who were out of the workforce, 60 percent, compared to Ely's 41.5 percent—indicating more retirees.[124] Incomes and housing costs are also higher outside Ely.[125] The demographic differences also coincided with political differences. In the 2016 election, Trump won 48.4 percent of the vote in Ely, compared to Clinton's 41.8 percent, while in surrounding Morse Township, Trump narrowly won by less than 1 percent, and in Fall Lake Township, Clinton won 49 percent to 43.9 percent.[126]

Mobilization among conservation and outdoor-recreation groups has centered on potential impacts to the BWCAW, including polluting the water of this popular fishing destination, loss of land for recreation, destruction of wildlife habitat, and degradation of the wilderness experience due to noise and light from a large industrial operation. Environmental groups, which work on broader environmental issues, are involved, but the opposition is spearheaded by conservationists and led by the Campaign to Save the Boundary Waters (CSBW), which is exclusively focused on halting Twin Metals' project and all mining in the

BWCAW watershed (largely ignoring PolyMet's project, which will be located outside the BWCAW watershed).

The CSBW was formed by Northeastern Minnesotans for Wilderness (NMW) in 2013 to coordinate efforts to protect the Boundary Waters from the harms associated with copper-nickel mining, in coalition with other conservation groups.[127] NMW is a small, grassroots conservation group run by a group of Ely-area volunteers on a shoestring budget. Longtime members told me that a good turnout for a board meeting used to be eight people. But now, as the CSBW has grown into a state and national campaign with a multimillion-dollar budget and a staff of professionals and experienced political campaigners, NMW board meetings are packed, and the CSBW is no longer run by the local organization. The campaign has formed a coalition including statewide and national environmental and conservation organizations including the Izaak Walton League, the Wilderness Society, and the Natural Resources Defense Council. The initiative to form the CSBW was led by Becky Rom, a retired lawyer involved in the national conservation movement who was active in earlier struggles to protect the BWCAW. Rom grew up in Ely, where her father owned a canoe outfitting company and was one of the leading figures advocating for protection of the BWCAW during the 1960s and '70s. Many environmental activists I spoke with credit the CSBW's success to Rom's leadership, fund-raising abilities, and strategies, though inevitably, tensions have arisen as the CSBW has grown beyond the local group of volunteers.

The CSBW uses a range of tactics to build political support and increase public awareness, particularly leveraging the federal protections for wilderness areas and the social and cultural importance of the BWCAW.[128] The group engages in regulatory decision-making by submitting technical comments, and it has hired scientists, economists, and other experts to conduct analyses of environmental and economic impacts. Its extensive public-relations campaign involves social media, op-eds, and events held around the state, such as a fund-raiser at microbrewery in Minneapolis and a film screening at a Patagonia store in St. Paul. Creatively, the CSBW organized several adventure advocacy trips to raise awareness and get media attention. These headline-making endeavors included a couple who paddled a canoe covered in petition signatures from Ely to Washington, DC, in 2014, then lived in the BWCAW for the entirety of 2016, documenting their adventure through a blog, book, and film.[129] A separate 501c(4) organization, the Boundary Waters Action Fund, was created to do the political work of lobbying, coordinating public petitions, getting out the vote, and endorsing politicians.

The CSBW has expanded beyond traditional environmental groups as it works to enlarge its base of support and appeal to more conservative and rural constituencies. Its coalition now includes Sportsmen for the Boundary Waters, created in 2015 to coordinate across hunting and fishing groups such as the Backcountry Hunters and Anglers. Another partner is the Boundary Waters Business Coalition, formed in 2017 and representing over two hundred businesses ranging from national outdoor-clothing companies, such as the North Face and REI, to local canoe outfitters to small regional businesses including breweries and coffee roasters.[130] These companies frame opposition to mining around the economic costs of pollution to outdoor recreation and tourism. Veterans for the Boundary Waters, also partnered with CSBW, argues that public lands and wilderness areas need to be protected as places of refuge for veterans in need of recreation and healing. This multifront effort has found some success. Even a few Twin Cities Republican politicians have begun to voice concerns about the Twin Metals project. That said, nearly all the politicians on the Iron Range, regardless of party, staunchly support the development.

Polling funded by the CSBW found that statewide opposition to mining near the BWCAW has increased, going from 62 percent in February 2015 to 67 percent in February 2016. But the CSBW's awareness and opposition-raising efforts have not spread to all copper-nickel mining; the public opposition is particularly aimed at mining *near the BWCAW*, such that only 28 percent of respondents in 2015 opposed copper-nickel mining *in Minnesota*, but 62 percent opposed it in the BWCAW.[131]

The supporters of Twin Metals, many of whom are also advocating for PolyMet's project and copper-nickel mining more broadly, insist that Twin Metals would bring jobs and economic development to a struggling rural economy. The company, industry groups, construction unions, and local politicians have stepped up their public-relations efforts to mobilize supporters and bolster political backing against the better-known efforts of the CSBW. The industry-labor coalition Jobs for Minnesotans has coordinated union members and local residents to attend hearings and held press conferences and rallies to support mining. Grassroots pro-mining groups springing up include Up North Jobs, Fight for Mining Minnesota, and Minnesota Miners. Though they coordinate with business groups, these organizations are not simply industry front groups or astroturfing operations; they formed through social media and personal networks. Iterations of the anti-federal wilderness groups that were active during the 1970s BWCAW conflicts, such as Conservationists with Common Sense, are also working with the pro-mining groups and connect with issues of promoting local control of land, weakening environmental regulations, and multiple use of public lands, encompassing motorized recreation, industrial activities, and conservation.

Shifting Politics and Prospects

The Twin Metals mine is a political football, with the likelihood of construction swinging back and forth depending on what party holds state and national political office. In 2016, the project appeared to be moribund. In March, Minnesota Governor Mark Dayton (DFL) declared that no state mineral leases within the BWCAW watershed would be sold or used for exploration and denied Twin Metals access to state lands.[132] This was largely a symbolic action: most of Twin Metals' mineral leases are federally owned and are underneath federal land in the Superior National Forest. Nonetheless, the governor's declaration created logistical barriers, since the company planned to use state lands during construction and operation.[133] Later, in December 2016, Twin Metals was dealt a more significant blow. The Obama administration revoked the company's federal mineral leases when they were up for review after expiring in 2014.[134] The USFS declined to renew the leases, citing "deep concerns" about potential environmental impacts to pristine waters in the BWCAW. The USFS and BLM then initiated an assessment of whether the leases should be eliminated outright, which meant soliciting public comments and holding a series of crowded public listening sessions in the Iron Range and Duluth.[135] On December 14, 2016, the leases were canceled. The agencies determined that copper-nickel mining did not coincide with management plans for the Superior National Forest and the BWCAW, since it posed an unacceptable risk to ecosystems, tourism, and tribal rights.[136] In announcing the decision, US Secretary of Agriculture Tom Vilsack said, "The Boundary Waters is a national treasure, special to the 150,000 who canoe, fish and recreate there each year, and is the economic life blood to local businesses that depend on a pristine natural resource."[137] The USFS went further, requesting that the US secretary of the interior enact a twenty-year mining moratorium on 234,000 acres of the Superior National Forest within the BWCAW watershed.[138] A two-year programmatic EIS on the effects of mining across the BWCAW was ordered to inform the decision on a twenty-year moratorium, which halted all mining exploration in the meantime.

Yet shifting political winds breathed new life into the Twin Metals project. The Republican Trump administration quickly reversed the Obama-era decisions upon inauguration, giving the project a new lease on life. Late in 2017, the BLM reinstated and renewed Twin Metals' federal mineral leases.[139] Then, in January 2018, the USFS reduced its EIS on mining in the BWCAW watershed to a less stringent process, an environmental assessment (EA), but even that was eventually suspended by Secretary of Agriculture Sonny Perdue.[140] The idea of a twenty-year moratorium on mining was dropped, giving companies the green light to move forward with mining proposals.[141] Twin Metals submitted its formal mine plan to state and federal agencies in late 2019, initiating the environmental review and permitting process.

Decisions to renew the Twin Metals project did not happen in a vacuum. A lobbying firm for Antofagasta and Twin Metals repeatedly met with top officials at the Department of the Interior to solicit their support.[142] Documents acquired by environmental organizations through Freedom of Information Act (FOIA) requests show that Antofagasta's CEO directly approached the then-secretary of the interior Ryan Zinke to request a meeting on Twin Metals.[143] Zinke, a former congressman from Montana, is a hunting, fishing, and recreation enthusiast, and some conservation and outdoor-recreation groups were initially optimistic when Trump picked him to lead the Department of Interior.[144] Once in office, though, Zinke and the Trump administration accelerated extractive development on federal land and wholeheartedly advanced the interests of the fossil fuel and mining industries.[145] The Trump administration quickly got to work making good on campaign promises to "Make America Great Again" by aggressively rolling back environmental protections, securing "energy dominance," and fast-tracking industrial projects. These moves included decisions to shrink the size of Bears Ears National Monument in Utah and approve construction of the Dakota Access Pipeline, both despite opposition from tribes and environmental groups.

Yet Twin Metals had not scored a touchdown. In 2020, the issue was punted back to a Democratic administration with the election of Joe Biden. The Biden administration reversed Trump-era actions, rescinding Twin Metals' federal mineral leases and restarting the environmental assessment of mining in the watershed of the BWCAW to inform a decision on a twenty-year mining moratorium.[146] In response, the MNDNR stopped work on a state-level EIS for the project.[147] Yet again, the Twin Metals project is on hold and in legal limbo. Even if future political maneuvers or lawsuits lead the company to get back its leases, permitting and construction would take years, if not decades, to complete.

Different Socioecologies of PolyMet and Twin Metals

The PolyMet and Twin Metals mines would extract the same type of metals and be located in the same region, yet there are important geographic, biophysical, and political differences between the two projects. The major difference is that the mines are in different watersheds, which has elicited different regulatory, political, and social responses. The two sites are only about twenty miles apart, but the NorthMet mine is a few miles south of the Laurentian Divide, which separates the St. Louis River watershed (feeding into Lake Superior) from the Rainy River watershed that flows through the BWCAW and into Hudson Bay in Canada. Thus, PolyMet's runoff, seepage, and leaks would probably not impact the BWCAW; Twin Metals' would.[148]

These geographic locations trigger different regulations and ecological concerns. The federal wilderness protections that apply to the BWCAW create additional regulatory scrutiny and pollution standards for Twin Metals. The potential moratorium on mining in the BWCAW watershed proposed by the Obama administration and restarted by the Biden administration is only possible because of the federal wilderness protections—which do not impact PolyMet. The St. Louis River watershed has less stringent protections than a federally designated wilderness area but also has a greater ability to mitigate the effects of acid mine drainage and is already impaired by industrial pollution, unlike the relatively pristine waters of the BWCAW.[149] However, there is more wild rice habitat downstream from the PolyMet site, which is a major concern for Ojibwe tribes.

The varying types of land and mineral ownership mean different levels of jurisdiction are involved in decision-making, which informs the strategies of opponents and supporters. The NorthMet site is on USFS land; thus, PolyMet needs to implement a land swap replacing the federal lands that would be destroyed by open-pit mining. Environmentalists have had some success in targeting that land swap with litigation. However, PolyMet owns private mineral leases, which means there is no requirement for public input on exercising those leases and little opportunity for lawsuits over the leases. Twin Metals, on the other hand, plans to lease federally owned mineral rights, meaning federal agencies make those decisions and need to solicit public input. Therefore, the projects' prospects depend heavily on who is in power in Washington, DC. Environmentalists have focused litigation and political pressure on renewal of Twin Metals' mineral leases, which has led to the project being delayed and potentially halted. However, since Twin Metals is proposing an underground mine, less land will be destroyed, and it does not need to trade land with the federal government or destroy extensive wetlands, unlike PolyMet.

Northern Minnesota's Iron Range is a place like any other, where local, historical, global, and contemporary factors all converge. Proposals by multinational corporations to mine copper and nickel have been controversial, even though the region faces economic struggles and an aging, decreasing population, making corporate promises of job creation enticing to some residents. Yet a slow transition away from an extractive economy and toward tourism and service industries also means that fewer people in the region have material connections to mining and that there are competing economic interests at play. In chapter 3, we will turn to the ways that different groups identify with this place and how that informs the perceptions and reactions to copper-nickel mining among both opponents and proponents.

3

Knowing the Land

Place and Emotion in Environmental Politics

The Tuesday Group organizes weekly luncheons at the Grand Ely Lodge, a resort, hotel, and event center on the shores of Shagawa Lake, just a few minutes' drive from downtown Ely, Minnesota. Invited speakers give presentations and lead discussions about a broad range of topics, from community issues to arts and crafts to science, for a crowd of regulars (many are retirees who relocated to enjoy nature and tend to be rather protective of the BWCAW) who snack on fried walleye sandwiches and burgers named the Paddler and the Camper. On, appropriately, a Tuesday afternoon in July 2017, attendance was particularly high. With every seat filled in the large conference space, people stood around the edges of the room—no one had time or space to eat. A leader from the Campaign to Save the Boundary Waters would present on the Twin Metals proposal and copper-nickel mining near the BWCAW. The controversial topic brought out a wider range of attendees, including mining supporters and longtime residents. People in "Save the Boundary Waters" gear sat alongside those sporting "We Support Mining" pins, and there was a level of tension and excitement that was rare at the Tuesday Group luncheons.

The CSBW representative opened with a concession. Humans need minerals and have been mining since the Stone Age, he said, and to his knowledge, no one affiliated with CSBW was anti-mining. Instead, the group opposed *this type of mining* in *this location*. When he said that copper-nickel mining was just too risky for the treasured BWCAW, I heard a sigh behind me. A white man in his fifties or sixties, wearing a pro-mining hat, muttered about "them not wanting it in their backyard." In the fight over copper-nickel mining on the Iron Range, it appeared groups were not so subtly contesting who could speak for the place and who could claim northeastern Minnesota as *their* backyard and to be representatives of the "people."

In this chapter, I explore why some groups support risky extractive development and how they frame their positions and claims to authority differently than the groups that are so adamantly against it. The conflict over copper-nickel mining is undoubtedly one involving place-based identity. It is about who can legitimately speak for the place, a struggle among different class-based and regional meanings of place, and divergent populist claims about letting the "people" make decisions and protecting US interests. Will mining development restore a nostalgic heyday of white, rural, masculine, and working-class prosperity while bolstering national security? Or will mining development hand over public lands to multinational corporations to make profits while leaving behind pollution, destroying the ability of future generations to enjoy clean water and tranquil wilderness? Cultural frameworks differing across class and region impact whether mining is seen as risky and out of place or safe and consistent with the place. Differences in groups' cultural frameworks lead to different interpretations of shared symbols like the land, mining, and outdoor recreation.[1] In order to garner support and spur action, different groups frame the issue to align with these frameworks.

Mining proponents see this region as a working industrial mining landscape, which has coexisted with clean water and outdoor recreation. They place trust in new technology and government oversight to ensure that copper-nickel mining is done safely and cleanly. Meanwhile, opponents see the mining landscape as toxic and a future to avoid—they do not share rural and working-class people's connection to mining. Opponents also distrust the ability of technology to make mining a "clean" industry. Yet, as white settlers lodge their appeals to place-based authority and being "insiders," Indigenous understandings of place are all but silenced, indicative of how industrial and wilderness projects alike have relied on rendering Indigenous presence invisible to construct land as "open" for white settlers to engage in masculine uses of resource extraction and adventurous outdoor recreation.[2]

Both mining opponents and proponents use dominant discourses of environmentalism, science, and masculinity to frame their positions and assert legitimacy and authority, contending that they are dedicated to protecting the local environment and that their position is supported by science. This is indicative of what the environmental and feminist scholar Sherilyn MacGregor calls the "masculinization" of the environmental movement, in which discourses of science and expertise take priority over political and moral claims.[3] Yet industry and its supporters have also taken on the rhetoric of environmentalism and sustainability through the discourse of ecomodern masculinity. Pro-mining groups and leaders, especially from unions and Democrats, argue that they care about the environment and that technology and economic growth will provide solutions to environmental problems. Mining copper, nickel, and other metals is said to be necessary for building the batteries, solar panels, and electrical wires required for creating renewable energy and transitioning to a more sustainable economy.

When opposition to hazardous industrial development is led by people of color and working-class communities, their efforts are often framed as *a struggle for justice*.[4] When it is led by wealthy, white communities blocking development near their property, it tends to be framed as a "not in my backyard" (NIMBY) defense of privilege.[5] By digging into the Iron Range's contention over a pair of proposed copper-nickel-mining sites, I challenge both of these framings. There are, in fact, many complexities and contradictions behind the ways different groups react to risky industrial development, especially when working-class residents raise "place it in my backyard" (PIMBY) demands, while middle-class people and those living further away push back. Place-based identities linked to mining are a powerful aspect of the ways industrial siting comes to be seen as natural, despite damage to the environment and exploitation of workers; place-based identities embedded in the exact same geography can also create resistance to extractive industries.

Opposition to copper-nickel mining is not neatly categorizable as environmental justice. There is internal division over what places and issues to prioritize: protection of wilderness, a typically white and upper-class priority, or public health and Indigenous communities. A mere twenty miles separate the Twin Metals and PolyMet sites, but they sit on the opposite sides of a watershed divide, which creates a cultural and political divide. Some opponents prioritize protecting wilderness and recreation areas, thus stopping Twin Metals within the watershed of the BWCAW. Yet other opponents think PolyMet should be a priority because it is in a watershed with larger downstream communities, including the Fond du Lac Reservation, a community that is already confronting health risks from the legacies of industrial pollution. Many of the mainstream environmental groups frame the issue through narrow conceptions of justice that fail to challenge systems of capitalism, settler colonialism, patriarchy, and racism that create ecological crises and socioeconomic dislocation.

Place-Based Mobilization

Communities often mobilize to defend a place against unwanted changes and perceived threats.[6] In Minnesota, this has meant white, working-class Iron Range residents and leaders mobilizing to support development as a way to defend their place-based mining way of life and urban and suburban middle-class environmentalists mobilizing against new mining projects that threaten their sense of place, whether it is wilderness or clean water. Copper-nickel-mining development is a struggle over what it means to protect the place, promote justice, and manage a landscape in which many people prize their labor, recreation, and heritage.

Lots of research has suggested that working-class, and often white and male, support for mining development stems from promised economic benefits, conservative politics, and corporate manipulation.[7] Yet, on the Iron Range, the motivations of longtime residents, community groups, and mining and construction unions appear more complex. I find that their PIMBY demands are shaped by a sense that new extractive development is a form of justice—a move that will protect their rural, white, masculine, and working-class moral economy and collective identity. Putting miners—an emblematic symbol of hypermasculine labor—back to work provides a way to strengthen hegemonic masculinity, which is perceived as threatened by the loss of traditional male breadwinner roles and a sense that elites and environmentalists disparage rural masculine practices like driving motorboats and ATVs and hunting. The feminist political ecology scholar Cara Daggett describes a similar dynamic in support for fossil fuels, in which extracting and burning fossil fuels is seen as central to white patriarchal ways of life that are threatened by climate change and economic crisis.[8] As Rebecca Scott reminds us in her research on coal mining in Appalachia, masculinities are not just important to men but also to broader communities, which, especially in extractive regions, are often defined by men's work.[9]

Support for new mining is not simply about the jobs. Many of the pro-mining activists are retirees, and some never worked in the mines; thus, they will not personally benefit from potential new jobs. Employment in mining has been shrinking for decades and, these days, represents only about 7 percent of regional employment. Those are largely male jobs; 92 percent of the region's miners are men.[10] The federal government in 1974 did force companies to hire women when nine of the country's largest steel companies signed a consent decree requiring that the industry's mines provide a share of new jobs to women and racial minorities. Still, women have never represented large numbers, and those who did enter Minnesota's iron mines faced rampant sexual harassment.[11] Yet today, many Iron Range women promote copper-nickel mining—indicative of how masculinities matter not just for men and are constructed in relationship to femininities. Left out in the dominant narrative repeated by regional political and business leaders and media are the many jobs in health care, social services, hospitality, and education that surpass the number of mining jobs and employ more women while also doing work necessary for the community's survival and well-being.

Further, the estimated number of jobs tied to the proposed mines is relatively small at the regional scale: around 350 full-time workers at the NorthMet mine and 700 at Twin Metals. Certainly, these jobs would benefit individual workers, yet many of these jobs are sure to go to skilled workers from outside the region. The sociologist Robert Wuthnow has written extensively about small towns and the US Midwest and finds that in rural areas, residents often take on community-based, rather than individual, perspectives to assess issues and therefore may support industrial development out of a sense that it will bring broader prosperity, regardless of any personal benefit.[12] Here, regional identities are strongly tied to mining. The Iron Range is like many rural landscapes, defined as working-class places by a labor history of mining, farming, ranching, and logging. This creates a sense of community identity linked to industry that extends beyond individual workers and those with direct experience in the industry.[13] Place and collective identities are intertwined with class identities and masculinities, and new mining may be seen as a way to strengthen the community and protect a moral economy built around male breadwinners working in extractive industries, regardless of whether individuals stand to benefit themselves.[14]

"We've been a mining area. This is how Ely got started," a retired teacher told me as he described growing up and then raising his own family in the town. Indeed, Ely is emblematic of how a place and collective class identity can be strongly defined by even a declining industry. There has not been an active mine in this town for over sixty years, but longtime residents maintain a sense of mining as culturally symbolic, part of a founding narrative in which the heroic hard work of male, immigrant miners built this rugged and remote region.

Pro-mining groups, mining corporations, and supportive local leaders are able to tap into emotionally salient place-based identities linked to mining to mobilize support and frame the projects as inextricable from the region's way of life. These voices are authorized through media coverage and statements from elected officials and respected community leaders as well as museums, memorials, and other official memory sites. Interestingly, the pro-mining argument is not framed using conservative ideals about individualism and property rights; instead, people describe their active support for the copper-nickel mines as a defense of their rural and working-class collective identity and a way to provide stable livelihoods to sustain the community. When I asked Randy, a community leader and DFL activist who retired from working in the iron mines, how he had been involved with the copper-nickel-mining issue, he began by recounting his union-member history and his family's connection to the industry. He felt that his work was like a calling, which was why he wanted more mining and the ability of future generations to follow in that calling. "I'm a third-generation miner, and a couple of my cousins, their kids are fourth-generation miners. It's in our blood. It's what we do." Mining is constructed as a naturalized identity linked to the community and family—a potent mix that leads people to equate protecting this emotionally salient mining-region identity with support for the arrival of copper-nickel mining.

I heard many longtime residents on the Iron Range talk about their towns being built by mining, implying that without mining, these towns and communities would lose their identity, even die out. At a crowded public hearing hosted by the US Forest Service in Duluth, a popular DFL state representative from Ely gave an impassioned statement favoring the Twin Metals project in which he reminded the crowd that Ely existed because of miners and could not live on tourists' money alone. When I asked Roberta, a white woman in her forties who is the mayor of a small town, why town governments, business organizations, and residents were supportive of copper-nickel mining, she described mining as being integral to their way of life and something they knew and trusted: "It's a mining town. The mine built the town. The houses were all steel: steel sidings, steel windows, steel garages. Everything was steel. So, yeah, it's literally a mining town."

This dominant narrative presents mining as the lifeblood of the community. It silences negative aspects of that same history—the dangerous and exploitative working conditions in iron mines and industrial pollution—in favor of the idea that copper-nickel mining might lead to a resurrection, helping this rural, industrial region regain its footing amid decline.

Residents of rural extractive regions may support development, even accept pollution, when industry taps into these emotional place-based, masculine, and class identities to frame development as *protecting the community*.[15] Meanwhile, *environmental protections* are interpreted as a collective threat that undermines the community's identity and moral values.[16] Appeals to place-based identities and a sense of community, which are very strong in rural areas, are increasingly important for sustaining the legitimacy of an industry that has growing environmental risks and decreasing material benefits. In *Removing Mountains*, the sociologist Rebecca Scott finds that Appalachian residents support mountaintop removal coal mining, despite the devastating environmental consequences and few jobs, out of a desire to defend the moralities of working-class masculinities tied to being self-sufficient breadwinners.[17]

A Place for Outdoor Recreation and Wilderness

Meanings of place are not monolithic. Contested and complex, this place-making in rural areas can mean that people find a sense of place seated in outdoor recreation, natural splendor, and clean water.[18] This can spark opposition to industrial development. When a place is identified with wilderness and experienced through recreation, industrial development may be interpreted as a threat.[19]

In Minnesota, critics of Twin Metals' proposed mine, largely white, middle-class residents who live in suburban and urban areas, frame mining as out of place and a risk to the Land of 10,000 Lakes—a popular slogan that is emblazoned on Minnesota license plates. For conservation, outdoor-recreation, and tourism groups involved with the Campaign to Save the Boundary Waters, the group described in chapter 2 that is focused exclusively on fighting Twin Metals and protecting the BWCAW, the project is understood as a threat to public lands and a rupture to experiences of tranquility in wilderness. The group frames opposition through *wilderness populism* to present mining companies as threatening the people's right to use and enjoy the land. Populism has long been present in US conservation discourse, as founders like Gifford Pinchot and John Muir talked about protecting national treasures and creating recreation opportunities for the American people. However, their vision of the "people" was racialized, classed, and gendered, as historians and social scientists have shown that many of these mainstream conservationists valorized a middle-class and masculine way of enjoying nature through recreation and adventure—some even had ties to the eugenics movement.[20]

People associate the area near the Twin Metals site with boating on nearby Birch Lake or setting off on a canoe trip via the Kawishiwi River, which abuts the mine site. Ely, recall, has not had an active mine since 1967; and so the Twin Metals site is also farther away from the existing mining landscape, and the surrounding area is largely forested. On a summer afternoon, I met a young staff member of the CSBW for a canoe tour of the area. Before launching our boats into the Kawishiwi River, just a few minutes of paddling from the boundary of the BWCAW, we stopped at a Twin Metals test-drilling site. The small patch of gravel was just a few hundred feet off a public road into the Superior National Forest that I could easily drive on in my Prius sedan. Down the road was a US Forest Service campsite and the popular Voyageur Outward Bound School.

Environmental advocates in the Ely area were concerned that Twin Metals would bring other development and industrialization, compounding disruptions to their experience of a serene and beautiful place. For example, Roger, who retired and moved to Ely, gave a very NIMBY-esque summation: "We don't wanna live in the middle of heavy industry. So, even if—I would not want to see it happen. I don't think it's appropriate." Julian, another Ely-based environmentalist, said, "My biggest fear is thinking of this incredible jam of monster trucks on the highway." A mine could meet every environmental regulation and use all the best available pollution-control technologies, but it would still be a rupture to Roger and Julian's shared vision of the place, on the basis of the traffic and noise alone—the same humming engines and thumping truck beds that, to mining advocates, sing of economic activity that is the community's lifeblood.

CSBW activists charge that copper-nickel mining is too risky for this cherished place. To them, northeastern Minnesota's landscape should be experienced through canoeing, camping, and other forms of recreation that maintain an idyllic vision of wilderness. Because of their class and residency, these often-white-collar professionals have collective identities tied not to mining but to a place seen as beautiful but now threatened. They have spent time in the region during summer camps and family vacations or even relocated to the area to live nearer forests and lakes. Ecofeminists argue that aspects of this desire to protect nature and keep it untrammeled by humans reflects masculine and patriarchal ideologies in which nature is seen as separate from society and in need of rational control and protection.[21]

Dennis is an active volunteer with the CSBW, and I met him at the organization's office in a small house on the main street in downtown Ely on a weekday morning in the summer—the busy tourism season, when the CSBW office, dubbed "Sustainable Ely," serves as an information center for visitors. Dennis had a legal career in the Twin Cities and spent much of his free time at his vacation home just outside Ely, canoeing and exploring the woods. When he and his wife retired, they moved up north full-time. Dennis has become very involved in efforts to stop Twin Metals. I inquired about the experience of moving to Ely and why the area was important to him: "I love wild country, and this [BWCAW] is one of the great, intact, more or less, wild ecosystems in North America, in the United States certainly. I love wildlife. I love the idea that there are places that are relatively uninfluenced by current human activity, where the flora and fauna can find their own way, as it were, by and large." These affective dynamics of place—the love for the BWCAW—are powerful in mobilizing action.

The CSBW launched what one leader described as a "value-based campaign," or an emotional and moral framing that effectively connected to collective identities tied to the BWCAW. I asked Todd, an owner of a canoe-guiding company, why he got publicly involved with the CSBW and endorsed the campaign as a business owner. He began by describing an obligation to defend the place and was poetic as he spoke of the natural environment in this region: "On a real emotional level, I think [it] is important for the people who visit here [BWCAW]. It can be a real life-changing experience. . . . It's just unique. There's no place like it." To mobilize supporters and generate public support, the CSBW's communications strategies could leverage this emotional angle, explained Mark, a volunteer and a retired professor in his sixties who lived in Ely, during an interview, when I asked him about what types of messaging were effective: "Well, I think you start with sense of place. That is just very powerful with the BWCAW. I mean that so many people have visited the BWCAW and even those that haven't just recognize it as a very special place and deserving of protection. I think that is the sell." As the sociologist Kari Norgaard affirms, this is an effective approach: appeals to romantic notions of nature can provide moral and emotional justifications for a group's position.[22] This emotional resonance helped give legitimacy to mining critics' claims. The wilderness populism discourse helped secure legitimacy and emotional resonance among a largely middle- and upper-class and white constituency outside the Iron Range, for whom the BWCAW carries strong cultural symbolism. Public hearings about Twin Metals held in St. Paul attracted thousands of people, while fund-raisers held by the CSBW at a microbrewery and Patagonia store in Minneapolis pulled in large crowds—few of these types of events were held in Ely.

Canoeing is an important cultural symbol for this opposition group. The CSBW even used a Wenonah canoe—a popular, Minnesota-made brand—nicknamed "Sig" (in honor of the conservationist and nature writer Sig Olson) as an eye-catching prop in its petition campaign against copper-nickel mining. When I stopped at the CSBW's booth at the Minnesota State Fair in summer 2017—where "Sig" was on display—one of the half-dozen volunteers, a white woman in her twenties, quickly approached to ask whether I had ever taken a canoe trip in the BWCAW. We talked briefly about canoeing, before the volunteer pivoted to the threat posed by copper-nickel mining. This pitch relied on my experience with wilderness recreation—a pitch that presumes a white, middle-class target audience (and, for this volunteer, that seemed appropriate in approaching me).

In the same way Minnesotans describe mining as a proud heritage and essential way of life, residents can also present connection to the outdoors as an essential component of being a Minnesotan. Brad is white and in his twenties and moved from the East Coast to Minnesota, where he started working as an organizer for the CSBW. During our conversation at the organization's office in a refurbished warehouse in Minneapolis, he reflected on what drew him to Minnesota and to get involved in environmentalism: "There's also this outdoor legacy [in Minnesota], this nature that people here just go out and explore and take to the woods and take to the canoes and take to the rivers and streams. And they utilize their outdoor space so efficiently and so beautifully that it's just part of being here." The focus on recreation has enabled the CSBW to expand its coalition to include hunting and fishing groups, outdoor-gear companies, and tourism businesses that want to protect the iconic BWCAW but are not *necessarily* concerned about broader environmental and political issues.

This framing has its blind spots, as well. Wilderness recreation is a specifically white, middle-class way of relating to the land that might not carry the same resonance for the Iron Range's white and rural working class, Indigenous people in the northern reaches of the state, or Somali refugees living in Minneapolis, even though all of these groups enjoy the environment and outdoors in various ways. When these activists envision a place separate from humans and society, that renders labor and Indigenous people invisible, a particularly problematic turn in a place populated and used by Indigenous peoples for millennia and impacted by centuries of commercial and industrial uses. It is a flaw common to conservation arguments; the earliest American conservation figures, like John Muir, tended to speak of nature as a place for healthful leisure and spiritual reflection, not labor and livelihoods.[23] The idea of wilderness as a place devoid of human occupants reproduces a myth that this land was empty and untouched by humans, lacking civilization and land management prior to European arrival.[24] When conservationists frame work as destroying pristine nature, it also ignores how labor can *also* be a meaningful way to engage with nonhuman nature.[25]

When Indigenous people *are* depicted, it is often in the context of a long-gone era, not as fellow residents. An environmental activist described the BWCAW in a *New York Times* op-ed article this way: "Today this region, the Boundary Waters Canoe Area Wilderness, looks almost exactly as it appeared 10,000 years ago when Paleo-Indians lived there."[26] Dating the landscape to time immemorial—at least, prehistoric time—again leaves out the ways it has been shaped by human activity, by *Indigenous* activity and presence that continues in the present day.

In my conversations, I rarely heard about the class, race, and gender dynamics of wilderness. Deborah's interview was an exception. She is a white woman in her fifties and a staff member of the Friends of the Boundary Waters, which is active in the struggles over PolyMet and Twin Metals. She acknowledged that rhetoric about wilderness was typically directed at white and upper-class people, and she pointed out that there are different ways of relating to nonhuman nature. She described a diversity initiative that her organization is leading to expand access to wilderness recreation: "We're hoping to be changed as well, that we maybe understand nature and wilderness from different cultural perspectives that will help inform the way we message, the way we do our outreach, to be more relevant, more inclusive." Her critical reflection was an outlier in my research, especially in contrast to the CSBW's messaging, which shied away from race, class, and indigeneity.

Clean Water and Public Health

Yet even mining critics are divided over what places should be prioritized for protection, which leads to different strategies and framings. This divergence is seen in the politics around PolyMet and Twin Metals. Although the projects are only about twenty miles apart, a watershed divide changes how they are understood. PolyMet is on the south side of the Laurentian Divide, where potential water pollution would flow not into the BWCAW but into the St. Louis River and Lake Superior. The PolyMet site is associated with the already industrialized Iron Range landscape, as it is near operating iron mines and would reuse an old taconite-mining facility. The St. Louis River watershed is already contaminated from decades of industrial development, particularly these iron-ore mines, so many of the lakes and streams have elevated levels of toxins, like mercury, and deteriorated fish and aquatic plant populations.[27] Since 1987, the US EPA has listed the St. Louis River among its forty-three Areas of Concern (AOCs) in the Great Lakes.[28] Much of the land is currently inaccessible—I was only able to get inside the fences and observe the mine site during an open-house tour offered by PolyMet—and it is not actively used for recreation.

For all these reasons, the CSBW's leaders made a strategic decision to focus on blocking Twin Metals. It seemed like, with the symbolic power of the BWCAW and the legal protections due to its status as a federal wilderness area, it would be easier to gain public and political support. The CSBW further justifies its Twin Metals focus by pointing to PolyMet's greater political support (including from Democrats), owing to its proximity to other mines and distance from the bulk of the tourism industry. I asked Elliot, a white CSBW staffer in his thirties who was living in Ely, about the differences between Twin Metals and PolyMet, and he described how the Twin Metals location was an evocative target for activism: "We're lucky, but also, we were unfortunate how close it [Twin Metals' mine] is to the wilderness area. It's just your charismatic megaphone that you're saying the Wild Life Foundation used to get donor money. You start to get less attention with PolyMet that is down by other lakes, and it could pollute Lake Superior." According to him, without the social resonance of the BWCAW, fund-raising and convincing the public to oppose the project would be far more difficult if the group was trying to stop PolyMet.

In contrast, groups that are working to oppose PolyMet argue that it is equally important as opposing the Twin Metals project, if not more so; PolyMet is further in development and may pose greater threats to environmental justice and public health. For these groups, the already polluted landscape is a reason to focus on stopping yet another hazardous industrial project that would increase the pollution burden on downstream ecosystems and residents, including Indigenous communities. Instead of the wilderness framing, they talk about risks to clean water, public health, and taxpayers. These different priorities and strategies have created some tensions among environmentalists, paralleling the long-running conflicts over race, class, and indigeneity within the US environmental movement. Here, mainstream and conservation-focused organizations have different priorities, strategies, and constituencies than environmental justice groups do.

Different priorities among environmental groups reflect different social valuations of landscapes. The area potentially impacted by PolyMet is not necessarily of less value ecologically than the area near Twin Metals is, but it is not as frequently used by white recreationists and tourists. Therefore, the area does not carry the same cultural meaning as the BWCAW. However, the land that PolyMet would transform into an open-pit mine is undeveloped and designated as an area of high biodiversity significance (despite the pollution), boasting abundant habitat for rare and threatened species and native plants.[29] Thousands of acres of ecologically important wetlands would be destroyed by the mine.

Many of the largest and oldest environmental organizations in Minnesota have joined with a handful of grassroots environmental groups to take a holistic approach to copper-nickel mining in which all proposals are viewed as intertwined, inseparable from all other mining projects. They point to the many people at risk living downstream from PolyMet in Duluth and Cloquet and on the Fond du Lac Reservation. Doctors and nurses raise urgent public health concerns about its potential to disproportionately impact the health of rural, low-income, and Indigenous people, as well as women and children. Groups working on PolyMet prioritize it strategically, knowing that it is closer to approval than Twin Metals is and that its approval as the state's first copper-nickel mine would set a precedent. To build a bulwark against the normalization of copper-nickel mining in this region, PolyMet's opposition is working to hold the project to the strictest standards or, potentially, stop it altogether.

Groups active on PolyMet frame the project around threats to human health and clean water, corporate accountability, and financial risks to taxpayers, rather than wilderness and recreation. Charles is a sixty-something white man who works for the Minnesota chapter of the Izaak Walton League, a prominent national conservation organization. I asked him why the group, which has historically focused on outdoor recreation, conservation, and protecting the BWCAW, was involved with both Twin Metals and PolyMet. Fighting both projects, he said, was necessary but involved using different messaging and targeting different audiences: "It's no question to us. It's not about just the Boundary Waters. That is something that—let's put it from a national perspective, where we send out national alert—that's probably well-known to our members who live in Maryland or something like that, whereas they wouldn't know where the hundred-mile swamp is or where the St. Louis River or even Duluth perhaps."

Ojibwe bands have also focused on PolyMet. In part, this is because they have a formal role in the environmental review and permitting process, which, as of spring 2022, was on hold for Twin Metals after having its federal mineral leases canceled. While I cannot claim any knowledge of the tribe's internal strategies or political decisions, there are major risks to the Fond du Lac reservation and 1854 Treaty territory raised by the PolyMet mine. PolyMet's threats to the well-being of Indigenous peoples and tribal rights are equal to, if not greater than, Twin Metals'. The St. Louis River watershed (*Chi-gamii-ziibi* in Ojibwe) has been the homeland of the Fond du Lac Band for millennia, a culturally and historically important place for which, the tribe claims, the PolyMet mine would be an "existential threat."[30] Water pollution or a tailings dam collapse would devastate the downstream reservation, but even normal operation would disrupt a Tribal Historic District studded with trails, canoe routes, villages, trading posts, and hunting camps, as well as traditional subsistence practices like sugar bush and wild rice harvesting. A factsheet created by the Fond du Lac and other Ojibwe bands explains that these ancestral places and historical uses are important, whether or not the lands are currently being used: "Religious and cultural importance to Indian Tribes is not tied to continual or physical use of that place. If an area remains in the hearts and minds of tribal members then that place is significant."[31]

Wild rice is a powerful symbolic food native to Minnesota, and scientists and tribal resource managers have carefully detailed how areas downstream of PolyMet are known for wild rice harvesting, regardless of its gradual depletion owing to existing industrial pollution, development, and climate change.[32] Additional pollution from PolyMet, in the form of sulfate releases and leeching heavy metals, would put further stress on wild rice and increase already-elevated mercury levels, rendering fish toxic for human consumption and further harming Ojibwe subsistence. Should these impacts harm wild rice and fish harvests for the Fond Du Lac Band's members, it would probably violate treaty rights.

The BWCAW, on the other hand, has less wild rice habitat and is used by Ojibwe people for hunting and fishing less frequently than the St. Louis River watershed is. Restrictions on using and accessing wilderness areas, regardless of the fact that tribal members are exempted from certain wilderness regulations, are further disincentives, contributing to long-standing conflicts between Ojibwe members and white conservationists and sportsmen over treaty rights in the BWCAW.[33] Thus, the priority of the primarily white and middle-class CSBW to stop mining near the BWCAW does not align with the concerns and efforts of Ojibwe tribes and Indigenous activists. Different priorities, cultures, and understandings of nonhuman nature have contributed to fraught and tenuous relationships between non-Indigenous environmentalists and Indigenous communities in Minnesota that look a great deal like conflicts throughout the US.[34]

Josh, a white man in his forties who has worked for a variety of environmental organizations in Minnesota, met me for an interview at a coffee shop in St. Paul. When I asked him about whether his organization had worked with tribes or Indigenous groups, he reflected on this tense history and the culpability of white environmentalists: "There's a long history of, frankly, really problematic relationships between Eurocentric environmental groups and the tribes. And so it's been a long process of building trust." Those who are trying to repair relations point to Indigenous activists and environmentalists whose shared interests have led to the building of successful coalitions opposing US pipelines and mining projects.[35] Similar alliances are possible in Minnesota, and, indeed, they are emerging around the PolyMet project.

There are a few environmental organizations in Minnesota that are active in opposing PolyMet and work in solidarity with Indigenous communities. WaterLegacy, a grassroots group that is led primarily by white people but includes some Indigenous leaders, is among them. Unlike most other environmental groups, WaterLegacy foregrounds tribal sovereignty and treaty rights. Its critique of copper-nickel mining highlights environmental justice, public health, Indigenous rights, and corporate accountability. A factsheet it produced regarding the PolyMet project includes the following: "The PolyMet mine site would be located on Treaty lands, where Lake Superior Chippewa retain rights to hunt, fish, and gather. Negative impacts of the PolyMet mine on wetlands, fish, plants, and wildlife would disproportionately affect Ceded Territory and downstream tribal resources. Rights to fish and hunt for subsistence are core values to Minnesota's Ojibwe Bands and is a part of their cultural identity."[36]

Friends of the Boundary Waters is also just starting to collaborate with tribes. Josh, a staff member of the organization, described how it tries to follow the lead of tribes, which play a key role in environmental regulation given their status as sovereign nations: "If anything, the tribes, especially in the state of Minnesota and especially Fond du Lac, deserve an incredible amount of credit. They have literally built a water-quality program that is the equivalent of a state program from the ground up in the last decade. So we work with the tribes and share information with them, but we never assume that we are dictating strategy to them. We want to take our lead from them as much as possible." Josh recognizes that tribes are nations that have their own regulations and governments, and he expresses a sense of humility and deference to their rights and expertise.

Tensions among Environmental Groups

The different responses to PolyMet and Twin Metals have generated some conflict between and within environmental organizations. Several of my interviewees who were working for groups active on PolyMet claimed that separating opposition to these two proposals played into industry's strategy since dividing the issue could weaken the opposition. Separating the issue into two discrete mines created an opportunity for Democratic, and even a few Republican, politicians to juggle critique and support of mining in an attempt to balance competing demands from labor unions and environmentalists. For example, Minnesota Democrats including the governor, Tim Walz, and both US senators signaled approval for PolyMet while raising objections to Twin Metals. The CSBW's silence on PolyMet gave politicians cover: they could support PolyMet and construction and mining unions while also working with the CSBW to fight Twin Metals and support environmental protection.

Josh, the environmental organization staffer I introduced earlier, felt strongly that focusing on Twin Metals was essentially sacrificing

Lake Superior and PolyMet's downstream communities to protect the BWCAW. When I asked him about the different strategies and priorities of environmental groups, he described some tensions while insisting that both projects needed to be addressed: "There's serious disagreement in the environmental community about this approach. Everyone wants to see the Boundary Waters protected. But I also wasn't willing to say that that also means that you can sacrifice the other side of the Laurentian Divide, and the people who live downstream are bad." His comment points to a fundamental consideration throughout the environmental movement in this country: Should they focus on protecting human populations or wilderness and recreation? Environmental justice groups specifically charge that mainstream and conservation-focused groups have not prioritized protecting people, particularly marginalized communities.[37]

Mark, a volunteer with the small Northeastern Minnesotans for Wilderness group, from which the larger CSBW grew, acknowledged that the group's ability to raise funds and attract public opposition through appeals to wilderness appreciation had created tensions with environmental groups working broadly on copper-nickel mining. When describing the CSBW's messaging, he remarked, "And that makes some other environmental groups unhappy because they think the BWCAW is getting special protection and feels itself deserving of special protection. And the fact is, it is. That is what the law says." He is not wrong—the Boundary Waters are insulated by stronger legal protections than other areas of the state are—though his comment does not address the need to navigate differences in political strategy and priorities.

Organizations are also complex. I found a variety of opinions among staff and volunteers involved with the CSBW. Several thought that increased scrutiny on Twin Metals would lead to increased public concern about copper-nickel mining and thus increase scrutiny on PolyMet. It was not that they supported PolyMet's construction but that they thought focusing on Twin Metals was the best public-relations strategy. Organizational leaders and lower-level employees and volunteers sometimes disagreed on this point. For example, some CSBW volunteers actively opposed both mines and saw the leaders' Twin Metals–focused strategy as shortsighted. Roger, a retiree now living in Ely, saw this as a sticking point in his volunteer work with CSBW: "The campaign

[CSBW] doesn't want to talk about PolyMet. And I think it's very important to talk about PolyMet. First of all, we used to live in Duluth; we love Duluth. And Duluth is downstream. Second of all, if PolyMet gets the go, it'll make it easier for the next mine and the next mine and the next mine to get the go. So the precedent's set." Roger does not like the thought of Duluth becoming a sacrifice zone for PolyMet in order to get Twin Metals' project shelved.

Contested Meanings of the Landscape

The physical landscape of the Iron Range has been transformed by a century of mining. As you drive up from the flat terrain of central and southern Minnesota, a ridge of hills is your first hint of the leftovers: massive pits and heaps of tailings and overburden. These, in other words, are piles of rocks left over from iron-mining operations. And class and regional cultural frameworks mean that different groups see the very landscape differently: many longtime Iron Range residents and mine workers see this mining landscape as part of their everyday experience, which is consistent with outdoor recreation and a symbol of economic

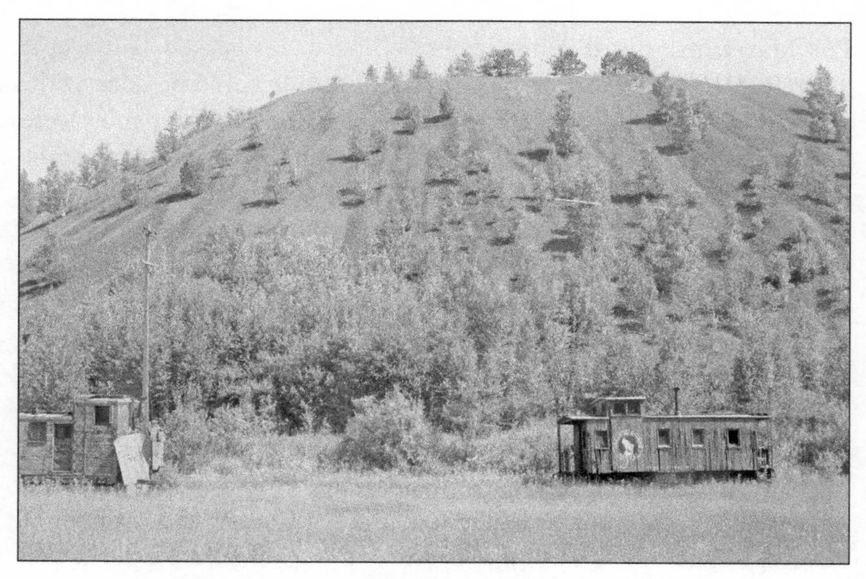

Pile of tailings from iron-ore mining. (Photo by Erik Kojola)

prosperity and technological prowess. Mine opponents tend to see the mining landscape a symbol of industrial destruction and pollution that is out of step with their vision for the place.

Marty is a retired teacher and informal community leader in Ely and met me for an interview at one of the two coffee shops in Ely. During our conversation, I asked him whether he trusted the ability of regulators and company officials to ensure that copper-nickel mining was done safely. He felt that government agencies would uphold their responsibilities and wanted to impress on me how well iron-mining companies had done in reclaiming former sites so that they were attractive recreation destinations:

> I think mining companies for the most part have pretty much done a good job of that [cleanup and reclamation]. I take a ride through the Range now, and you see a lot of your big ore old dump areas there. They got trees going up in there, and it actually looks pretty decent, some of them like mountains. I just think here at our Miner's Lake right here, that was the old Pioneer Mine there. There are trout basically in that lake that are probably as lively as any place and very abundant. That goes to show you that those things can happen.

For Marty, mining did not leave behind a devastated landscape. Therefore, he believed that copper-nickel mining could be done without long-term environmental degradation, so long as companies were held accountable. His perception, however, required overlooking some important facts: reclaimed mining landscapes often lack a healthy and diverse ecosystem, and copper-nickel mining is more hazardous to water sources than iron mining is. Any future copper-nickel-mine pit lakes would be highly toxic, with water too acidic for safe swimming, fishing, or drinking, more similar to the headline-grabbing reclaimed Berkeley Pit in Butte, Montana, where thousands of migratory snow geese died when they landed on the acidic water.[38]

The same landscape that Marty sees as a proud example of safe mining, the prowess of labor and technology, and reclaimed recreation is interpreted by environmentalists and conservationists as a scarred industrial wasteland—a harbinger of worse things, should copper-nickel mining be approved. Brad, a young, white CSBW staffer who recently moved to Minnesota, sounded very different from Marty when he told me about the operating and reclaimed mine pits he had seen: "When you get to that overlook around Virginia [Minnesota], you can see the giant pits from a height. . . . It's crazy. It's these gigantic, open, pits. That's what all of this is. And you can see some of them filling with rusty-orange water. I personally wouldn't swim in that." Despite being open to public use, including swimming, these iron-tinged mine pit lakes are, to Brad, a symbol of industrial toxicity. Sandra is an older white woman who grew up in Ely and recently moved back after living in the Twin Cities for much of her adult life and is now among the most prominent leaders of the CSBW. She told me that Twin Metals would "take out a huge swath of national forest land immediately adjacent to the wilderness. It would look like the Mesabi Iron Range." To her, the Iron Range beyond the BWCAW is a landscape to be avoided, not celebrated.

The cultural and political importance of clean water and outdoor recreation leads both sides to frame themselves as protecting the place that they know through time spent on lakes and rivers. Yet, how people spend their time in nature fractures along class and rural-urban differences in outdoor-recreation culture. Different forms of recreation, whether its hand fishing ("noodling," in local terms) versus fly fishing, or bird watching versus bird hunting, carry strong meanings of class, masculinity, and place identity.[39] The US conservation movement has a history of viewing how rural and working-class people relate to nature as backward and uneducated and a threat to wilderness, unlike upper-class forms of outdoor leisure.[40] Meanwhile, working-class rural residents have come to resent the restrictions imposed by conservation policies and the perception of being judged by outside elites.

Class and rural-urban tensions over outdoor recreation have played out acutely in Ely. One of the biggest divisions is over motorboats and canoes. The 1978 Boundary Waters Canoe Area Wilderness Act banned motor-vehicle use in much of the area, reserving it for nonmotorized recreation. For many longtime residents, this action was seen as privileging middle-class and urbanite ways of experiencing nature: hiking, canoeing, and cross-country skiing. There are lingering resentments about outsiders constraining the ability of locals to enjoy the place by using motorboats, ATVs, and snowmobiles, which are forms of recreation popular among working-class and rural residents. The BWCAW itself is taken as a symbol of the imposition of outside forces on the Iron Range—a limitation on locals' rights and overreach by the federal government.

Boating, fishing, hunting, and other popular outdoor recreation activities are part of the Iron Ranger identity that spans all political stripes. While paddling on Burnside Lake—a large lake near Ely that is outside the BWCAW—on a gorgeous sunny afternoon, I spotted a lakefront house with a "Mining Supports Us and We Support Mining" sign. This is the same lake where the famed conservationist and nature writer Sig Olson's cabin and twenty-three-acre retreat—Listening Point—is located and now preserved as a memorial and site for environmental education.

I was struck by mine supporters' use of outdoor-recreation rhetoric and expressions of concern for a clean environment. The dominance of lakes, clean water, and outdoor recreation in Minnesota culture means that pro-mining groups frequently make claims to environmental stewardship. Mine supporters reconcile outdoorsmen identities with the threat of water pollution from copper-nickel mining by emphasizing their experiences with iron mining as a clean industry and their expectation that copper-nickel mining will also be safe. They regularly referred to the use of flooded iron-mine pits for swimming, fishing, and boating (one, called Miner's Lake, is just a few blocks from downtown Ely and is stocked for trout fishing, although I had no luck catching any). They pointed to the Mesabi Trail, a bike path weaving through 135 miles of fields and forest dotted with piles of waste rock.

A number of environmentalists hoped that mutual appreciation for clean lakes and rivers and outdoor recreation could create common ground with pro-mining folks. Todd, the CSBW activist and guide-company owner, expressed these sentiments when I asked him about the potential for bringing together opponents and proponents of mining: "I think people really appreciate the outdoors up here and kind of the wilderness area and the fishing. It's really important to people, and it's kind of their sense of self. So I think that's common ground. . . . I think most people would say, if they thought this mine would pollute the Boundary Waters, they wouldn't think it was a good idea." His comment highlights that key divergence: whether or not people think copper-nickel mining can be done safely.

The CSBW has expanded to include sportsmen's groups, outdoor-recreation companies, and small businesses, diversifying the coalition beyond traditional environmental and conservation groups. These efforts to connect with groups representing more conservative, rural, and working-class constituencies have done little to build local bridges, however; some of the sportsmen's groups are actually national organizations. This strategy has failed to be transformative, in part, because local supporters believe, or at least publicly claim, that copper-nickel mining can be done safely, but it also hinges on deeply engrained social and cultural divides. Mine opponents frame conservation and a rejection of new mining around wilderness, tranquility, and canoeing, which does not resonate with the ways Iron Rangers connect to the land. The hunting and angling groups opposed to Twin Metals are proponents of low-tech recreation—using canoes and backpacking to access remote areas, rather than motorboats and ATVs—which is often framed as being an upper-class way of experiencing nature. Iron Rangers largely write off this rhetoric and these groups as still reflecting elitists and outsiders.

Yet some BWCAW-motivated mining opponents suggested that their counterparts were resentful about regulations and did not actually appreciate the wilderness area. When I asked Elliot, at the CSBW, about his interactions with people in Ely, he brought up the different recreation cultures and contrasted going into the BWCAW in a canoe, getting off grid, with locals' ideas about enjoying nature:

> There's still that resentment in town, even with kids my age. I'm thirty, and I've got good friends my age who have never been onto a Boundary Waters lake other than Basswood Lake, and they've lived here their entire lives. There's just that resentment from their family: "I don't want to go on a paddle trip. What the hell, no. Let's just go to Bass Wood in a motor boat and put a big old tent and party for a week and catch a bunch of fish." It's still there. It's bred into, and it's really hard to go against that.

His words reveal a social and cultural divide over the wilderness and the sense that "they" hand down disregard for the natural world, generation after generation. His account draws on cultural tropes about backward "rednecks" that naturalize rural people as deviant. It is not a particularly generous statement, though Elliot clearly felt strongly as we talked.

Who Has a Right to Make Decisions?

Groups struggle over authenticity, legitimacy, and claims to being the best stewards of the land. They contest who is "local," who can claim this place as their "backyard," and in turn, who has a right to speak for the place. Both sides make populist claims about democratic and just decision-making and speaking up for the people and the land and water, but based on different concepts of who constitutes the "people," what publics are affected by these decisions, and how to best protect the place. This reflects how struggles over land are often about competing notions of justice and who can claim the right to make decisions. How these voices become authorized and amplified is shaped by political-economic and cultural power. What groups can fund active public-relations campaigns? What voices do politicians listen to? And how do claims resonate with broader cultural narratives and symbols? Concern for a clean environment has also become common sense such that all sides argue that their position will protect the environment. Pro-mining groups turn environmental arguments against opponents, claiming that they are selfish NIMBies and that copper-nickel mining is actually green since it will provide metals necessary for renewable energy production and be done in a place with strong environmental laws.

It's Our Backyard

The rhetoric of extractive populism (more on this in chapter 5) dominated the public comment hearings that I attended, in which pro-mining speakers proudly claimed to be third- and fourth-generation Rangers, asserting their deep connection to and right to decide what is done with the land as well as commitment to protecting clean water and air. Iron Rangers, like residents of other rural places, have intimate knowledge about the environment where they live that is passed on through generations and created through hands-on experience recreating and working on the land.[41] This also means that they frame the possibility of mine development being blocked by the government or environmentalists—outsiders and elites—as an injustice violating locals' moral economy and right to determine how their backyard is used and to create prosperity from extracting natural resources. Politicians from northern Minnesota and business leaders evoked these arguments in their public statements, giving them added authority and volume.

Mine supporters frame opponents as urban environmentalists who could not truly know, and in turn protect, the place. This reflects a theme in which rural residents see environmentalists as out of touch with the environment, in contrast to their commonsense and everyday engagement with the land.[42] Research from around the US finds that rural people express pride in having close connections to nature and, as Loka Ashwood shows, assert higher moral standing than urban people, who are supposedly disconnected from nature.[43] This sentiment reflects what Michael Bell calls a "natural conscience," in which rural people view themselves as being more closely connected to the nonhuman environment through their daily lives and labor compared to urban people.[44] I asked Randy, the retired miner living in Ely, about his perception of mine opponents. He described them as dilettantes and lacking intimate knowledge about northern Minnesota's land and waters: "They [mining opponents and wilderness supporters] have a concept, some of them, that they just want to know it's here. They've never been here. I asked one girl—I knew that she wasn't very wilderness oriented—'Well, how many lakes have you been on in the Boundary Waters?' She said, 'All of them.' I said, 'Oh really?' I said, 'Name me a dozen.' She couldn't name three of them." Randy scoffed at ill-informed outsiders' hypocrisy and contrasted it with the locals who actually know and care for the BWCAW because it is where they live (and make their livings). Some Iron Rangers even claimed that these outsiders are an environmental problem in and of themselves, leaving trash in the wilderness and overusing campsites in ways that show they do not cherish the landscape like the locals.

Iron Rangers were angry about their perceived portrayal by mining opponents as unconcerned about the environment. Instead, local pro-mining groups and activists claimed that they are stewards of the place who care for the environment and asserted their moral superiority as people who care for the land. In my conversations and in public statements, people often recounted stories of spending their spare time hunting, fishing, and riding snowmobiles and ATVs, activities that they argued coexisted with iron mining. I was connected with Jerry through another person I met while living in Ely, and he invited me over to his house for an interview—he was happy to chat with a young, white graduate student. Jerry has lived around the Midwest, but in retirement, he and his wife picked Hoyt Lakes as an affordable and relaxing place to live. Jerry has blended into the local community, such as meeting a group of old-timers—many retired miners and all men—for coffee at the local diner most mornings. He invited his neighbor Tim, a retired miner who was born in Hoyt Lakes, to join us for the conversation on their patio. After his wife brought us glasses of lemonade, the two men told me about why they support copper-nickel mining and expressed being judged by mining opponents while asserting that local residents care deeply about the environment. Jerry put it this way: "You would get the impression, I think, when you go to these meetings that the people on the Range have no concern about the environment. That's a bunch of bologna. The people on the Range are the biggest bunch of hunters, fishermen, outdoor people . . . and are so concerned with all that kind of stuff. The last thing they want to do is ruin these lakes."

At a pro-mining rally, Democratic state senator David Tomassoni declared, "We know how to take care of our own backyard. We're not about to let anyone screw up our water or our air." In fact, mine supporters claim that they have kept the region so pristine that tourists flock here from across the state and country—all this as it functioned as a hub of iron mining for well over a century. The wilderness area that others say they want to protect, this argument goes, is the result of Iron Rangers' sensible environmentalism, not environmentalists' ideological extremism.

The boundaries between locals and outsiders are social constructions—they are made up, essentially, in ways that serve political ends. There are people living in northeastern Minnesota who oppose copper-nickel mining, but they may not be seen as "locals" if they were not born and raised in the region. There are people involved with environmental and conservation groups who have moved to the Arrowhead, particularly the area around Ely, in retirement or to start small businesses, yet they certainly now think of themselves as locals. In Duluth, the nearest city to the Iron Range, there are strong environmental organizations, but they, too, are framed by Iron Rangers as urbanites, outsiders—anything but "locals." Even the primarily northern Minnesota members of smaller environmental organizations such as

Northeastern Minnesotans for Wilderness and WaterLegacy are often denied local status, in part because their activism places them outside the dominant construction of who counts as an Iron Ranger.

When white descendants of European immigrants on the Iron Range claim that they are the true "locals" who can speak for the place, they are erasing those who came before and continue to live alongside them. These claims to a form of *settler indigeneity* naturalize the presence of white European descendants in this Native American landscape. Equating longtime rural white residents who have worked in extractive industries with Indigenous people is a discourse used in other natural resource conflicts to assert authentic connections to place and a right to use the land, while silencing Indigenous dispossession and colonial violence.[45]

Longtime residents' pride in protecting the environment, rhetorical or not, tends to tidily brush off the essential role of outside forces in ensuring environmental protection. Without state and federal regulations, Iron Range residents would have little recourse to influence and monitor corporate practices in their backyard. The environmental regulations that pro-mining groups claim already keep the environment clean were enacted largely through pressure from environmental activists and against the wishes of business. Further, the mining industry has tremendous influence on state politics, and new mining projects may translate into more political power for industry to weaken regulatory standards and enforcement.

Pro-mining groups flip NIMBY to charge that mining opponents are selfish NIMBies who do not want to risk their "playground" but are not dealing with the pollution in their *actual* backyards. They point to the polluted waters near the Twin Cities to argue that urban environmentalists are hypocrites who need to mind their own backyards. Steve, a pro-mining activist who owns a canoe- and fishing-guide company near Ely, quickly brought up critiques of environmentalists during our conversation and said mockingly, "I'm more of an environmentalist than they are. I don't live in the Twin Cities, where I put green stuff to make my lawn green, so my neighbors think it's pretty. . . . And I don't dump motor oil in the ground, and we don't do things that create eco-disasters." Urban lifestyles are framed as the actual environmental threat, in contrast to rural lifestyles and livelihoods that are deeply connected to the land through everyday experiences.

An extension of this line of reasoning also accuses copper-nickel opponents of pushing mining into more vulnerable people's backyards—to poorer countries lacking environmental and labor protections. A white male in his sixties warned me, for instance, that it would be stupid not to mine in Minnesota, because then it will be done in places like China, where mines pollute and employ child workers. Using similar language, Roberta, the white, forty-something mayor of a small Iron Range town, talked about environmentalists being hypocrites because they try to block PolyMet while accepting dangerous mining overseas: "Why is it okay for China to be killing ten thousand people a day because they have no environmental standards?" To her, it was narrow-minded and selfish to oppose Twin Metals and PolyMet: "They [mine opponents] don't care about the overall environment. I have the perception that they just want to have this as their own area."

The spurious claim that environmental opposition to mining in the US causes poor working conditions and pollution in the Global South tidily erases the culpability of corporate cost-cutting strategies and weak free-trade agreements. Constructing a mine in Minnesota also will not stop dirty and dangerous mining in other places. Using China as a symbol for the problems of globalization and a scapegoat for deindustrialization in the US ignores that China has never been a major producer of copper and nickel. Together, these statements reflect American nationalism and anti-Chinese rhetoric that have long circulated in US politics across the left and the right (more on these implications in chapter 5).

Another way that mine supporters argue that environmentalists are hypocritical and irrational is by raising the idea of green energy. "How," they ask, "will you get the copper needed for renewable energy and hybrid car technologies without mining that copper?" The logic goes: to transition to a greener economy, copper mining is necessary; therefore, copper mining should move forward in Minnesota with strong environmental regulations, labor standards, and a unionized workforce that, with its vested interest in the land, will speak out about pollution. (Recycling and lowering consumption, among other possibilities, are left unmentioned.) This rhetoric also reflects a shift away from hypermasculinity that celebrates industrial progress and domination of nature toward what Jonas Anshelm and Martin Hultman call "eco-modern masculinity," which mixes toughness with care for environment, often through technological and market solutions.[46]

Alex, a white construction-union staff member, was adamant in pointing out environmentalists' contradictions and told me,

> Nobody is saying, "Stop using copper." Nobody is saying, "Let's boycott copper." They're saying it's [mining has] never been done safely. But they're not taking the next step to saying, "Therefore we shouldn't use copper." Because you can't transition from a fossil-fuel-based economy to a renewable-energy-based economy without a shit-ton of copper. It is a necessary component in transitioning away from fossil fuels, which we [his labor union] support. If the question is not "Should we or should we not use copper?" then the question must be "Where and under what circumstances should copper be mined?"

Once again, seizing on environmental talking points about green energy allows pro-mining groups to frame themselves as more concerned about environmental issues than are mining opponents, who just want to protect their playground. The frequent mentions of clean and sustainable mining are indicative of industry appropriating the language of environmentalism, using claims of environmental and social justice to defend extractive capitalist development, and diffusing those logics to policy makers and receptive locals.[47] Roopali Phadke describes the contradictions between the resource needs of renewable energy and the ecological impacts of extracting those materials as the "green energy bargain."[48]

It's Everyone's Backyard

Environmental and conservation groups deploy *wilderness populism* to assert their own deep knowledge and stewardship of this landscape and critique foreign multinational corporations that want to extract value from the land while leaving behind contamination. The land, they argue (without, as was discussed earlier, much thought to the problems of settler colonialism), belongs to the public, so it is not only nearby residents who have a right to make decisions about its use. Mining opponents challenge that they are "outsiders," on the grounds that this place is *everyone's* backyard and that extractive development by multinational corporations is an injustice that creates profits for the *real* outsiders, international companies that care little about polluting this treasured place. However, appeals to protect wilderness for "all Americans" can overlook the class, race, and gender dynamics regarding who can and does use wilderness areas and the ways that appeals to the people are often implicitly white and middle class.

Groups focused on opposing Twin Metals frame themselves as having a right and a duty to speak for this place that they know so intimately by canoeing, hiking, camping, and otherwise experiencing the landscape. Bill is a white outdoor-recreation guide in his late thirties who has done trips to promote the CSBW. He described this perspective and his motivation for activism: "We see ourselves as just sort of bearing witness to this place, you know, and just being a constant reminder of how special it is and why we need to protect it." The CSBW regularly employs the religiously inflected language of "bearing witness" and positions the land as fragile and in need of protection by humans by speaking for "this quiet place." According to this logic, conservationists' reverence for non-human nature gives them the authority and moral obligation to defend the land against destructive industries.

Mining critics also challenge the argument that nearby residents should have greater authority in decisions about land use. They contend that the mines are on federal and state lands and that water and air pollution would have impacts across and beyond the region, which means these decisions are not local at all. Those who are focused on Twin Metals emphasize how the BWCAW is a national treasure enjoyed by people from all over the country and use the rhetoric of wilderness populism to contend that all US residents should have a say in its use. Sandra, the CSBW leader I introduced earlier, remarked in our interview, "This place belongs to all of America."

Conclusion

A kaleidoscope of class, race, and regional cultural frameworks have led the proposals for copper-nickel mining on Minnesota's Iron Range to be understood differently by different groups. These frameworks shape how people interpret the potential impacts of the PolyMet and Twin

Metals mines as threatening or strengthening their sense of place and how they work to frame their positions as legitimate and authentic.

The issue is a struggle over who can speak for the place and who can enact their vision for the landscape—an industrial mining landscape or wilderness recreation landscape. Supporters see proposed mining as renewing their sense of place and collective identity—as Iron Rangers in a productive industrial landscape—and argue that they have a right to determine how their backyard is used and that they are best situated to protect the water, air, and forests. Environmentalists and conservation groups view copper-nickel mining as too risky for a cherished national wilderness area and for the waterways that characterize Minnesota. They see this entire landscape as belonging to the public—as *everyone's backyard*—and use rhetoric of wilderness populism to argue that decisions about its use cannot be limited to the input of just nearby residents.

The cultural and political power of outdoor recreation in northern Minnesota means that both sides frame their position as aligned with the true character of the place. Mining advocates claim that they are the true environmental stewards of the place who have a deep knowledge of the environment and would not let their backyard be polluted. Industry and its supporters adopt environmental rhetoric to greenwash mining and frame opponents as hypocrites and NIMBies who are willing to accept pollution in other parts of the world to protect their playground. They argue that mining in Minnesota is actually key for sustainability because it will supply metals for renewable energy and other green technologies and will be done in a place with strong environmental regulations. On the other side, environmental groups claim that copper-nickel mining is inconsistent with the sky-blue waters of northern Minnesota and a threat to wilderness areas as well as downstream communities.

A look at the place-based identities and appeals in Minnesota's copper-nickel-mining case offers three key conclusions. First, meanings of place are important in the cultural frameworks people use to understand issues and the framing that groups use to mobilize support around contentious environmental issues. PIMBY demands for risky extractive development are based not only on material interests, the political-economic power of industry, or corporate manipulation but also on the ideological power of everyday cultural understandings and emotional connections to a mining identity and a sense of place intertwined with resource extraction.[49] Pro-development messages resonate as authentic when they connect with collective identities and emotional ties to a place dominated by extractive capitalism. As Eric Hobsbawm argues, sense of place is something actively created for political and ideological ends and is most effective when it appears as natural and timeless.[50]

Second, place identities are important in shaping the contradictions and complexities of interpreting notions of justice around hazardous industrial development. Perceptions of environmental justice depend on how people interpret social and environmental conditions as injustices or not.[51] In rural regions and working-class communities, expansion of hazardous industries can be understood as promoting justice, and blocking development can be understood as an injustice that denies locals the right to jobs and to determine how their backyard is used. Different interpretations of place can lead other social groups to view extractive development as an injustice, though if those groups live farther away or hail from the middle and upper classes, they are not necessarily at the highest risk of such injustice. As Stephanie Malin argues, it is important to understand the ideologies and dynamics of capitalism that shape how people come to hold contradictory views such as supporting risky industrial development alongside concern for the environment.[52]

Third, cultural and material factors are intertwined in shaping how groups understand environmental issues and engage in contentious politics.[53] Nature and society are coconstituted, and "natural" resources are the product of historical contingencies, sociocultural definitions, and biophysical properties.[54] We see this mutual constitution at play in Minnesota, where the chemistry of different types of rocks and minerals and hydrology of different mining locations lead to divergent political and social responses. Environmental groups frame copper-nickel mining as out of place, since it would be riskier than existing iron-ore mines due to the mineral composition of the rocks, which creates more risk of acid mine drainage. And while the PolyMet and Twin Metals sites are only twenty miles apart, they are in different watersheds, and this, too, leads to different political responses based on the social meanings of the different landscapes. Groups dedicated to conservation and outdoor recreation—which are largely white and middle class—focus on Twin Metals as a wilderness threat, while other environmental groups and tribes focus on the risk from PolyMet to downstream communities. These divergent priorities reflect political, racial, and class tensions found throughout the modern environmental movement.

4

Mining Memories

The Mobilizing Power of Nostalgia and Hope

The Pioneer Mine opened in Ely in 1888, one of the first iron mines in northeastern Minnesota. Over the next fifty years, mining boomed, transforming the rural Iron Range region into one of the world's largest producers of iron. Trains connected the region to Lake Superior ports in Duluth, where massive loads of ore were dumped onto barges that brought iron to steel mills across the Midwest and East Coast. But with booms come busts, and on April Fool's Day in 1967, newspaper headlines announced the abrupt closure of the Pioneer Mine. Sadly this was not a joke but rather the end of mining in Ely. Today, a group of former miners and community members are working to document the town's mining history and preserve some of the original buildings, structures, and equipment from Ely-area iron mines, including the Pioneer, that are now rusting and lie in disrepair.

A small museum run by a local nonprofit now operates in the old Pioneer Mine shaft house, providing an attraction for tourists and local history buffs a few afternoons per week (summer months only). The building's metal tower can be spotted from the edge of downtown and sits a few hundred yards from the flooded mine pit that is now called Miner's Lake. I visited the museum on a Tuesday afternoon in the summer of 2017. My volunteer tour guide was a septuagenarian white man wearing blue jeans, a work shirt, and leather boots who told me he had worked in the mine back in the 1950s and '60s. He showed me around the old mine shaft building and displays of black-and-white photos of workers throughout the years, of the mine site during its construction and in its heyday. As he explained how different pieces of mining equipment were used, emphasizing how technological advancements made it easier and faster to extract ore, my guide wove in personal stories of his time at the Pioneer—a good union job, he said, especially for a young guy who wanted to work hard. Its closure came as a shock to him, as it did to all the workers—the whole town, really. Many people moved away, with some relocating to work in other Iron Range mines. Those who stayed—like my guide—struggled to find new jobs. They had never done anything else. Toward the end of our tour, unprompted, he mentioned that Twin Metals was doing mineral exploration in the area. It would be copper-nickel mining, not iron mining, he pointed out, but he thought it could renew Ely's mining history, opening a new chapter for the region.

Several months later, I would hear other vivid accounts of life "up north" that warned against the vision that former miner embraced. Hundreds crowded into a microbrewery in a refurbished Minneapolis warehouse for a fund-raising event and book release, hosted by the Campaign to Save the Boundary Waters. When I entered, guests were perusing silent auction tables, sipping on craft beer as they mulled over prizes that included canoe gear and watercolor paintings of northern Minnesota scenery. Eventually, CSBW staff addressed the crowd, recounting their own experiences canoeing and fishing in the BWCAW—a special place that their organization wanted to protect from copper-nickel mining. Then they introduced Dave and Amy Freeman, well-known wilderness adventurers and recreation guides who, with CSBW sponsorship, had lived in the BWCAW for a year. The book that this event celebrated, as well as a short film, had come out of their experience, and the Freemans spoke passionately of their love for the pristine wilderness and unique landscape (even through a harsh winter in the woods and the summer's swarms of mosquitoes and vicious blackflies). They told the appreciative crowd that they wanted to preserve this incredible resource for future generations and that they hoped their book and documentary would "speak loudly for this quiet place."

These interactions highlighted, for me, the importance of emotional collective memories in animating conflicts over copper-nickel mining. Arguments at the grocery store and in town-hall meetings are part of a struggle over the region's past, present, and future, in which mining supporters and ardent detractors alike mobilize emotion and memory to give authenticity and legitimacy to their claims. Nostalgia and hope inform how different groups assess the impacts of potentially hazardous industrial development, leading to divergent perceptions of risks and benefits.[1] Romantic "smokestack nostalgia" for the heyday of mining and rural masculinity energizes pro-mining action and helps generate trust in corporate and state assurances of safe mining, abundant jobs, and a renewed era of prosperity.[2] Idyllic wilderness nostalgia anchored in the BWCAW is paired by some environmental and conservation groups with fearsome visions of a future, industrialized landscape devoid of family vacations and backcountry canoe adventures. Other groups, ones that are active on all copper-nickel-mining projects (including the Poly-Met project, which would be outside the BWCAW watershed), rely on appeals to the future, contrasting the incredibly long time horizon of pollution's deleterious effects with the clean water needed to support future generations. In both of these contrasting collective memories and future imaginaries, we see the complex progressive and reactionary potential for nostalgia and the ways it silences parts of history, whether its Indigenous dispossession or a male-dominated extractive economy, while also motivating people to fight for what they see as a just future.

Understanding why decisions about natural resource and land use become contested and generate passionate responses requires looking at people's emotional connections to place, anchored in the ways they remember the past and imagine the future. The concept of timescapes is useful; these cultural frameworks organize how people understand time and give meaning to the past, present, and future.[3] Collective memories, or shared narratives recounting the past, making sense of the present, and constructing possible futures, are key to timescapes, in that they help people remember their own experiences and relate to events outside their personal biographies yet within their relevant cultural frameworks.[4] The geographer Doreen Massey writes that "the identity of places is very much bound up with the histories which are told of them, how those histories are told, and which history turns out to be dominant."[5] The resulting social understandings coalesce into collective memories only through and following struggles over which histories and *whose* histories are remembered or forgotten. Collective memory can reveal who has (or once had) the power and legitimacy to represent the past and speak for the future.[6]

The past and future carry powerful emotional meanings, making timescapes crucial considerations for politics and social movements. Collective memories can motivate people to act, as emotions guide desires for the future, generate forward-thinking action (especially to defend land and livelihoods), and shape how different groups understand legitimacy and truth.[7] I focus on nostalgia, a nuanced form of memory that evokes longing for an idealized past, emotional attachments to place, and hope for creating a prosperous future.[8] The geographer Alastair Bonnett argues that nostalgia is adaptable to support both conservative and leftist movements.[9] Romantic, reactionary nostalgia is wielded by right-wing movements claiming to restore tradition (often the traditions of white supremacy and patriarchy) and also used to valorize histories of struggles for justice and resistance to advance leftist movements.[10] Nostalgia, in all its forms, tends to silence historical tensions, to leave out some portion of the larger story.

Throughout this chapter, I investigate the ways that different groups' timescapes are shaped by class, place, race (specifically whiteness), and gender, affecting their understandings of the potential risks and benefits of copper-nickel mining on the Iron Range and the legitimacy of competing claims. Both environmentalists and pro-industry groups use appeals to nostalgia as drivers of mobilization, but neither fits into neat boxes of progressive or reactionary, as both draw on hegemonic masculinities and tend to render Indigenous people invisible.

Competing Memories of Place

On the Iron Range, residents and community leaders yearn wistfully for the good old days of mining, leaving aside the ill health effects of industrial pollution, heteropatriarchy, and exploitative working conditions—what the sociologist Tim Strangleman calls "smokestack nostalgia," on the basis of his research with working-class communities experiencing deindustrialization.[11] In extractive regions, collective memories of masculine labor using brute force and massive machines to extract value from the earth necessarily inform how these places are defined in relation to industry.[12] Mining supporters hope that extracting copper and nickel will usher in a return to the good life—family-supporting wages, bustling downtowns, and packed stadiums at high school hockey games—without damaging their backyard.[13]

On the other hand, environmental groups that are opposed to Twin Metals use wilderness nostalgia to frame copper-nickel mining as a threat to collective memories of outdoor recreation and hopes for preserving the land and water for future generations to enjoy. Wistful yearning for the good old days of unspoiled wilderness also leaves aside a violent story of Indigenous dispossession that enabled creation of recreational wilderness areas and privileged access for settler tourists with the money and time for vacations. However, wilderness nostalgia is a less useful frame for critics of the PolyMet project, which poses less threat to outdoor recreation but greater risks to Indigenous communities, treaty-protected natural resources, and public health. In this conflict, we see the complex relationship American masculinity has with nonhuman nature—nature is something to control and destroy through technology and labor as well as something to protect and a place to demonstrate one's manliness through survival and adventure.[14]

Smokestack Nostalgia and Renewing the Mining Legacy

"Smokestack nostalgia" fits into a broader discourse of extractive populism (which I unpack in chapter 5).[15] It is a romantic collective memory that informs a hopeful vision of future prosperity ushered in by the development of a new type of mining. Social change often evokes this kind of yearning for a more prosperous and simplistic past, and so the closure of an industry that was key to a whole region spurs both a deep sense of loss, particularly for dominant masculinity centered around being a breadwinner and doing physical labor, and a keen desire for new industrial development that promises a future that looks like the past. Busts, like the one that followed the region's iron boom, give smokestack nostalgia its emotional power, and, as the scholars of memory Katharine Hodgkin and Susannah Radstone argue, that creates political power: how the past is remembered is key to how the future is imagined.[16] When mining is remembered through this variety of nostalgia, more mining is seen as the only way to breathe life back into dying mining towns, restore rural moral economies, and protect white and working-class masculinities tied to labor in extractive industries, constraining alternative imaginaries.[17]

In my conversations, Iron Range residents and local leaders regularly described their connections to the region's prosperous past—when mining provided white men with stable, family-supporting jobs. They shared fond memories about vibrant communities, back when mining jobs came with the good union wages and benefits that enabled the proverbial American Dream, including the luxury of leisure time, when workers and their families could enjoy the outdoors and be involved in the community. I was repeatedly told about the halcyon days when miners would leave their shift on a hot summer day, only to hop in a pickup truck and head to the nearby lake to go fishing (maybe to catch their family's supper). As I chatted in an Ely coffee shop with Rob, a middle-aged white man who grew up on the Iron Range, he told me how his personal and family histories were behind his activism in support of copper-nickel mining. Rob had not worked in the iron mines himself, yet he reflected on a time when there was more economic opportunity in the area, when men could easily get a good mining job without a college education: "A lot of the guys went right from high school, went right to the mines to work. It was that simple. You knew that when you graduated from high school that if you wanted a job, all you had to do was go into the human resources office at Reserve Mining or Minntac or wherever and go, 'I'm going to go to work.' They'll say, 'All right. We're going to put you on a production truck. Here you go.'" His comment reflects the dwindling prospects for decent-paying jobs, especially for workers without a college education, driven by deindustrialization and weakening of unions. Yet the romanticism overlooks the gender inequalities of the past and how women's roles were constrained and their fortunes tied to their husbands'. It also overlooks the environmental and occupational health consequences of mining, which carried a toll on miners' bodies and surrounding waterways.

Others spoke with pride about years past, when the local schools, built with mining royalties, were filled with students and fueled high school hockey rivalries, while main-street storefronts bustled. The retired miner Randy is an active community and political leader who suggested that we talk at Ely's Dairy Queen (a hangout that is popular with both retirees and high school students). After saying hello to a few other older men sipping coffee in the plastic booths, Randy settled into his family history. He told me how his grandparents had immigrated from Slovenia to work in the mines and about the prosperity he remembered from his own youth in Ely: "The youth are not here like there was when I was in school. And so back when I was growing up, we had like nine grocery stores in Ely. We had six women's clothing stores, five men's clothing stores. We had five car dealerships, and we had probably a half dozen, eight gas stations. . . . I mean, Ely had sixty-four hundred people about, versus thirty-four hundred and something now." The decline that Randy has lived through is now apparent in absences: jobs lost, kids moving away after high school, storefronts and gas stations shuttered. These daily reminders symbolize the region's struggles.

Mining and the immigrant workers from Europe who built the mines were presented as essential to the region's history by many others, too. Daniel, an Iron Range DFL state legislator in his early forties, also began our conversation with family history. We discussed his connections to union organizing and European ethnic food traditions, like his grandfather's pasties—the still-common meat-and-potato hand pies brought to the Iron Range by twentieth-century Cornish miners, then adapted by Italian immigrants, who added sausage, and Finnish immigrants, who tucked in rutabaga. When I asked Daniel to describe unions' stance on copper-nickel mining, he returned to the idea of mining as a part of the fabric of Iron Range life. To him, copper-nickel mining is less a union issue and more a "regional" issue: "People up here understand [mining] a little bit more just because we've been in the hotbed of mining for 135 years, and it's something we grew up with and understand very well, just like a farmer understands farming and factory-working areas understand manufacturing."

Aaron Brown, the Iron Range writer and Hibbing Community College instructor, writes of his homeland, "the memory of the 'old days' is fresh and often the currency of most conversations."[18] This was true in my experiences interviewing community and political leaders, who often became palpably more comfortable talking with me when they heard that my great-grandparents were Finnish immigrants and that my grandfather was raised in Hibbing and worked in the iron mines along with his brother. It was also apparent in the pride of people like my tour guide at the Pioneer Mine or Matt, an Iron Range city council representative and pro-mining activist, who prefaced our interview with a walk through his city hall's small museum. There, he pointed out faded black-and-white photographs of soot-covered men working in the iron mines and shoppers crowding downtown sidewalks. Then he took me outside to see the ornate carvings in the building's façade—"mining built all this," he beamed, and he hoped copper-nickel mining would be a legacy he could build for the next generation.

The companies aiming to open copper-nickel mines today appeal to this romantic nostalgia. PolyMet directly invokes the renewal of the good life and masculinity, claiming that the new mine "will continue the proud mining tradition on the Iron Range," which "has sustained tens of thousands of families, dozens of communities, schools, commerce and recreation centers."[19]

As research in other mining regions finds, collective memories of a mining heyday rely on an image of the heroic, proud, white, male breadwinner who could depend on the stability of his industrial job and his wife, working to keep house.[20] This vision of the "good life" blatantly ignores oppression of women, as well as labor exploitation and the hard-fought class struggles that made mining a decent job. Marty, a retired Ely schoolteacher, recalled that, growing up in the area, he had a dad who worked in an iron mine and a homemaker mom: "[My dad] was at the Pioneer Mine, and of course my mother, she didn't work. . . . My dad, he was a hard worker. He basically worked in the mine, and then on weekends, he would go out and cut pulp wood. That's a time when everything was done by hand, of course, with your crosscut saws. . . . He was a worker, I'll tell you. I don't know how he did it, but he kept going." In Marty's account, physically demanding work is remembered as a form of valiant masculine labor during simpler times, when men could make ends meet by working hard. It came as little surprise that Marty was cautiously optimistic about copper-nickel mining.

Some women did work in the iron mines, but not until the 1970s, when the federal government forced mining companies to hire women. The women who took jobs doing manual labor in the mines were some of the first women inside, and they faced rampant sexual harassment. Their landmark class-action sexual harassment lawsuit, *Jenson v. Eveleth Taconite*, was won in 1984 and chronicled in the book *Class Action: The Landmark Case That Changed Sexual Harassment Law* (adapted for the Woody Harrelson and Charlize Theron film *North Country*).[21] Smokestack nostalgia ignores pioneering women like Elizabeth, who was among the first women to work in the mines. She was in her sixties by the time of our conversation and recalled that she had spent eight years working at Reserve Mining. She only took the job to support her family and had few of the fond memories that male mining retirees shared: "I didn't like any part of it. I really didn't. It just was not something I ever wanted to do, and I thought, 'Okay, it might have been the best-paying job I'd ever had, might have had very good benefits, but I would never put myself through this experience again.' . . . In fact, of all the women that worked in the mines when I did, only one of them stayed with it afterwards. None of the rest of us would ever put ourselves through that again." Elizabeth had no romanticism for her mining job—despite the good pay—and the hardships she and other women endured. Yet this does not mean that Elizabeth opposed the industry. She was mildly supportive of the copper-nickel proposals and saw a need for jobs and economic development. This reflects how hegemonic masculinity also interacts with femininity and shapes how women understand gender roles and norms, particularly in tight-knit mining communities. R. W. Connell also argues that the construction of and contention over masculinity occurs at the personal and collective level, such that people's individual practices disrupting hegemonic masculinity may not be connected to structural and collective issues.[22]

There are alternative memories that recount the dangerous and demanding labor that went into iron mining. Randy, introduced earlier, recounted the harsh, dirty, and hazardous conditions:

> But [mining is] not always an easy job. It's a tough job. It's a dirty job sometimes. It's cold, hot. I mean, you go from one extreme to the other through the seasons. Even when you work inside, like, some of the plants in the basement, they're wet, water all over, muddy sometimes. You're crushing rock and everything to make powder, concentrates. Then you're baking that in a kiln at 2,450 degrees, and if we gotta go work on a crane and the kiln, because it's stalled or something, it's damn hot up there. . . . Main thing is be safe when you're working, watch what you're doing, watch out for your partner—it's like any job—if you want to come home the way you went to work and with all of your fingers and all of your toes.

Yet a dirty and risky job can also be a badge of masculine honor and pride—something not provided by jobs working in an office or retail store.

Pro-mining groups and local leaders decry the population loss in this region, implying that young people left because the mining industry left. They rarely acknowledge that the graying population is also due to people actively choosing not to go into mining and younger generations wanting a different lifestyle. Some younger people saw mining's dangers and physical demands, and they looked for something different. Chris grew up in Ely. Rather than follow his parents' generation into mining, he moved away and lived in Minneapolis, returning to the area in his forties, about a decade ago. He and his siblings, he explained, did not want the life their parents had: "Not wanting to do shift work, watching your dad go to work at eleven o'clock at night and get home at seven o'clock in the morning." Today he works at a local outdoor-clothing manufacturer and understands, but is frustrated by, the often-vehement defense of copper-nickel mining and the lack of alternative economic-development proposals.

With fewer and fewer Iron Rangers having direct connections to mining, it struck me as curious that the smokestack nostalgia remained so strong. Sure, there are active iron mines near some of the Range's western towns, like Virginia and Hibbing; but mining history is more distant in towns in the eastern part of the Iron Range, and fewer people work in the remaining facilities. Ely has not boasted an active mine in nearly sixty years. Yet people who never worked in mining still share the dominant community identities and collective memories that give mining corporations' proposals ideological power. Creating and maintaining the mining heritage identity is an ongoing process of struggle and politics, frequently constructed and literally cemented in the physical landscape, memorials, and museums, as well as in the media and political and corporate rhetoric.[23]

Museums are prime among the sites that place the mining industry at the heart of the community.[24] The Minnesota Discovery Center is the largest regional history museum, described by the historian Jeffrey Manuel as a focal point for nostalgic accounts of the Iron Range.[25] Originally formed as the Iron Range Interpretive Center in the late 1970s, it was intended as both a historical archive and an economy-boosting tourist attraction. It was built on top of an underground mine and next to an old mine pit. In 1986, the center was rebranded as Iron World and outfitted with elaborate, expanded displays on immigration and mining history; developers hoped it would bring a tourist renaissance to counter another economic downturn, but it, too, failed, closing in 2004. Its current iteration, the Minnesota Discovery Center, opened in 2006.[26] During my visit in 2017, the exhibits were focused on social and economic history, particularly immigration and mining, and geology of the region. The displays about mining often emphasized technical progress and the ingenuity of inventions that enabled miners to extract more materials. Exhibits about poor working conditions and labor organizing were presented as past struggles, and there was almost no mention of the industry's environmental impacts.

Several closed iron mines have been turned into state parks, complete with interpretive centers and guided tours. Here, too, I found the dominance of smokestack nostalgia. For example, I visited the Soudan Underground Mine State Park on a rainy Sunday afternoon in the summer of 2017. Soudan was the first iron mine in Minnesota when it opened in 1882, and it operated for eighty years. After it closed in 1962, the site was converted into a park and museum run by the Minnesota Department of Natural Resources. I parked my car and walked through the drizzle, passing old mine buildings and equipment on my way to the former mineshaft building, now the visitor's center. I signed up, along with several families and older couples, to take a tour down the old mine shaft and settled in to watch a short video about Soudan's history before we headed underground. The film opened in the 1950s, with a narrator calling Soudan "the Cadillac of underground mines." The voice continued as iconic '50s footage played: new cars being driven off dealer lots, bustling suburban shopping malls, and Elvis fans screaming at a concert. Then the film cut to interviews with proud former miners who spoke of the large amounts of iron ore pulled out of Soudan and how they formed a close family with their fellow workers. I could not help but notice that the film focused on the supposed heyday of mining and the prosperity that was enjoyed by white, male breadwinners throughout the US in that period, rather than on violent labor struggles in the early twentieth century or the downturn in mining during the 1960s that closed Soudan for good.

On another weekend afternoon, I visited the Hill Annex Mine—once an open-pit iron mine, it closed in 1978 and later became a state park, where you could tour the rusting remnants and learn about old mining trucks and excavators. As at the Pioneer Mine, this tour was led by

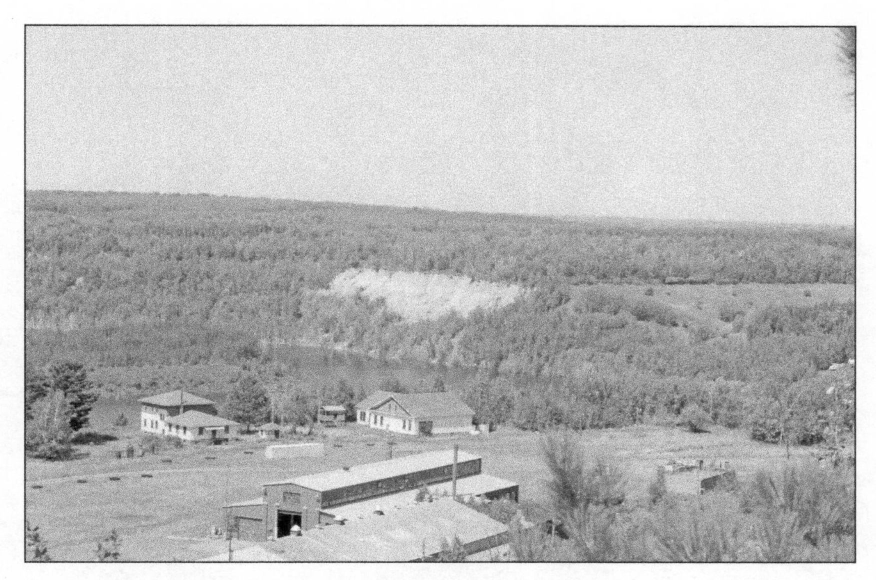

View of the Hill Annex iron mine that is now a state park. (Photo by Erik Kojola)

a seventy-something volunteer who was a retired miner. Wearing work overalls, he recounted story after story about working in the mines in his thick northern Minnesota accent as he drove us through the facility in an old school bus, stopping occasionally to let us explore old buildings and equipment up close. A few of his memories touched on harrowing accounts of near accidents, but most were about the benefits that he and his family members experienced working in various mines. In his stories, mining was a heroic, exciting job that was physically demanding *and* a way to make good money—he was still able to quote the exact wages and pensions that miners took home. During the tour presentation and his side conversations with tourists, I heard him talk about his hopes for the future of mining on the Iron Range. Whether it involved new technologies to extract valuable metals from old iron tailings or the proposed copper-nickel mines, he was in favor.

My travels brought me to many smaller memorial sites dotting the Iron Range landscape. Some stood at closed iron mines; others were simply civic commemorations. Along the highway, between the towns of Hibbing and Chisholm, I caught sight of an eighty-five-foot-tall statue of a miner, holding a shovel and pickax—the very image of the noble,

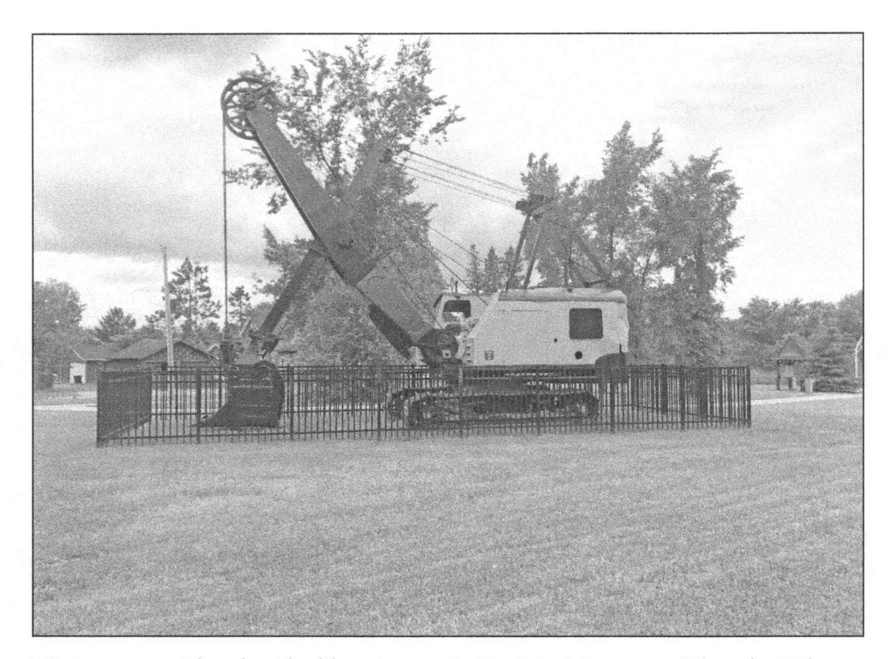

Mining memorial park with old equipment in Virginia, Minnesota. (Photo by Erik Kojola)

hardworking, male iron worker. The plaque below the towering copper and brass figure reads, "A tribute to the Mesabi, Vermilion, Cuyuna and Gogebic Ranges' men of steel, who carved out of a sylvan wilderness the iron ore that made America the industrial giant of the world. They shall live forever!" Other memorials make use of retired mining equipment and have plaques describing regional history and technical and geological details about mining operations. All of these displays celebrate the mining industry and the sacrifice of hardworking miners, reminding visitors that they built the region; many also embrace the technological advancements and bigger, more powerful machines that, ironically, sped the pace of the mines' depletion and displacement of workers.

Museums, memorial sites, and visitor centers are part of an effort to commodify mining heritage and shape the public's image of the industry. Interpretive signs and mine viewpoints are part of corporate public relations; the Iron Man statue I saw on my drive was paid for by mining companies, and many of the memorial plaques dutifully list the corporations that funded them. Presenting the industry as modern, clean, and essential to society means hewing to the narrative of progress, of extending a proud past into the future. The Minnesota Discovery Center, which began as a state-run project, is operated today by a private nonprofit and gets its funding primarily through mining-production taxes (administered by a state development agency, the Iron Range Resources and Rehabilitation Board [IRRRB]), public funding for arts and heritage, and corporate donations.[27] The center is currently a member of the Iron Mining Association of Minnesota, whose mission is to "promote the iron ore industry's long-term growth and prosperity."[28]

Beyond the dedicated sites, I uncovered mining history kept alive by the artifacts of active and former mines. Iron Rangers' are familiar, in their daily experiences, with the piles of rust-colored waste rock, flooded mine pits, and abandoned and operating mining infrastructure and buildings that evince mining heritage. In Ely, the old Pioneer mineshaft building is visible from downtown. My apartment during fieldwork was a few blocks from Miner's Lake, where I would take morning jogs

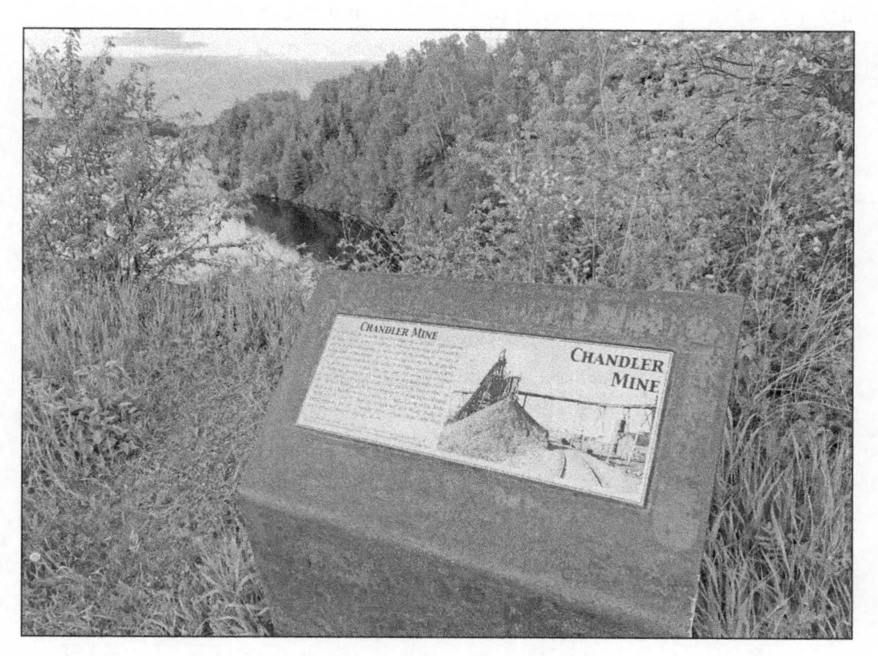

Plaque commemorating a shuttered iron mine along the Trezona Trail in Ely, Minnesota. (Photo by Erik Kojola)

around the Trezona Trail (named in honor of Chandler Iron Mine boss Charles Trezona). As I ran, I passed bronze plaques marking the mine shafts and buildings that once stood, as well as the current office of Twin Metals. There was a literal path that ran between mining's history and future.

For those who are more accustomed to reading than running down history, local media was a wealth of nostalgic collective memories. Regional newspapers, such as the *Ely Echo* and the *Mesabi Daily News*, regularly wove regional history into articles in favor of the copper-nickel-mining developments. A column called "Window into Yesterday" is a regular feature of the *Ely Echo*, and editorials and opinion pieces frequently invoke smokestack nostalgia (mostly to support the proposals). One *Ely Echo* editorial argued that Twin Metals should go forward because mining had already proven it could coexist alongside a clean environment: "[Locals would] like to be able to live, work and recreate here just as we have for over 130 years. Natural resource extraction has been going on here the whole time and yet by some miracle you can drink the water and eat the fish. Even out of a mine pit. Imagine that."[29]

There are still some alternative voices in the local press. Copper-nickel-mining opponents also write op-eds and letters to the editor, and there are a few publications that take a more neutral or skeptical stance on the issue. The main alternative voice comes from the *Timberjay*, a Tower-based paper that covers the greater Ely area, whose editor has written extensive investigative articles on the financial and environmental risks of copper-nickel mining.[30] It is clear that residents consider people's choice of newspaper as a political and social statement. In my experience, newer residents and environmentalists tend to read the *Timberjay* and sniff that the *Ely Echo* is a mouthpiece of the pro-mining factions. "Old Elyites" do the opposite, complaining that the *Timberjay* is nothing more than untrustworthy anti-mining rhetoric. I was well aware of the social signal I sent when I stood in line at the grocery store holding either a copy of the *Ely Echo* or the *Timberjay*.

Wilderness Nostalgia and Hopes for a Clean Future

Opposition to Twin Metals is framed through wilderness nostalgia—memories of childhood and family experiences with outdoor recreation, alongside hopes for a future in which others could continue to enjoy the clean, sky-blue waters of Minnesota. Wilderness nostalgia can be effective for mobilizing support for environmental causes as appeals to emotional memories of bucolic idylls can help make environmental issues tangible and salient.[31] The US conservation movement has long been motivated by nostalgic myths about the simplicity of a premodern world and getting back to nature through experiences in untrammeled wilderness.[32] A long-standing theme in American masculinity is that one can prove one's manhood through wilderness exploration and adventure.[33] In contrast, groups that are broadly active on copper-nickel mining issues, including on the PolyMet project, tend to eschew the wilderness nostalgia framing; they are not appealing to outdoor recreation and wilderness protection but to the uncertainties of new mines and technology and the risks of pollution to water and public health. They highlight the polluting history of iron mining and the need to protect natural resources, like wild rice and clean water, for future generations.

In my interviews, staff and volunteers with the CSBW often described their love for the area with the zeal of a first crush. They spoke of canoeing and camping in the BWCAW, of how it offered a place for social bonding. For example, Julian—a middle-aged white man who owns a small outdoor recreation and guiding business in Ely—cited his idyllic childhood memories as the reason he moved to Ely and became a leader with the CSBW:

> It was magical from the get-go [on a summer youth trip to the BWCAW]. The whole thing, from start to finish, was absolutely life changing. I remember it like it was yesterday. I still draw on it daily, memories of sunset evenings on an island in Basswood Lake, playing kick the can with my pioneer boy buddies and watching bear cubs camp around the far shore and listening to the loons and the sizzling of walleye filets on the frying pan over the campfire.... That riveting experience led me to set my sights on somehow, some way, calling this home someday.

The cultural symbols that Julian evoked are powerful for establishing a sense of place in this specific region: the unique call of loons (Minnesota's state bird, the waterfowl have a lovely, plaintive warble that travels over the water) and campfire-cooked and hand-caught walleye (the state's official fish, it has starred in many a church fish fry—as well as many of my parents' stories about their Minnesota upbringings).

Opponents of Twin Metals wanted to protect a cherished place that they remembered for their experiences of spiritual reflection and social connection. I met Johanna at her house near a lake a few minutes' drive outside Ely. She is in her early sixties and recently moved to Ely, where she can work remotely in her professional job while also finding the time to enjoy the outdoors. I asked Johanna why she got involved with the CSBW. Her response touched on copper-nickel-mining pollution being a threat to her cherished childhood memories and fear that others might miss out on this outdoor recreation experience: "I was going to live in this wilderness-edge community, where I was going to be able to do something that I loved that had been a part of my life since I was a teenager, and the idea that that was threatened was scary or an affront or certainly something that I should not just roll over and play dead [about]."

The BWCAW was presented by mine opponents as a place for self-discovery, tranquility, and respite from the stresses of modern life. Camping on a remote lake, only accessible by canoe, offered visitors the chance to listen to the sounds of insects, birds, and the wind without contamination from traffic and planes flying overhead and to gaze at the stars against a pitch-black background untainted by city lights. Many people described longing to get a break from their hectic lives and jobs and cherishing their time spent up north. However, the ability to "get away" is only accessible for those who can take vacations and pay for travel and equipment.

Environmental organizations strategically frame Twin Metals as a threat to these culturally and emotionally important memories. Another CSBW activist, Gary, had lived in Ely since the 1970s after moving there to work for a state agency. Now he runs an outdoor store and outfitting company that provides rental equipment and guides for BWCAW trips. When I asked why he thought the CSBW had been successful in raising public concern and convincing people to oppose Twin Metals, Gary pointed directly to emotional appeals: "Hundreds of thousands of people have been here over the years, and they don't forget it. This place influences more people emotionally. When you get an emotional tie to a place, you've got a real strong hold on those people." Perhaps the clearest example of wilderness nostalgia rhetoric that I saw came in an op-ed written by an environmental activist for the *Duluth News Tribune*: "Traveling by canoe and getting off lakes by mid-afternoon, we move slowly enough to see and hear things. A beaver swimming by as we play cards on a granite outcrop. A baby loon riding on its parent's back. A pine marten climbing in the tree as we read in our hammocks. . . . As I plan an August trip to the Boundary Waters, after a decade doing summer backpack trips in the Sierra Nevada, these memories flood back."[34] Painting a sepia-toned picture of the wilderness helps make the mining issue meaningful and emotionally salient.

The nostalgia that I encountered in northern Minnesota was less masculine than in other places, like stories about rugged men scaling mountains or risky backcountry downhill skiing in the western US, and often centered around family and appreciation for the nonhuman environment. This sentiment was on display at the 2017 Great American Canoe Festival held in Ely. I went to a literature event where authors read excerpts from their short stories, memoirs, and novels that were set in northern Minnesota. One presenter, a white man in his sixties, read a story about taking his teenage daughters on their first overnight canoe trip into the BWCAW. He reflected on how the challenging experience of hauling boats and heavy gear over long portages (when you have to walk between lakes that are not connected by water) and enduring bug bites from the swarms of mosquitoes helped his daughters mature and brought them closer together as a family.

Still, the collective memory of opponents of Twin Metals is a selective representation of the past. Descriptions of a pristine wilderness untouched by humans and outside of modern industrial society are partial, constructed narratives that rely on rendering Indigenous use of the land invisible. The ecosystem of the BWCAW has been shaped by human activity. Anishinaabe and other Indigenous peoples have used the region for thousands of years, actively managing the land, hunting, and harvesting plants. The region was used by voyageurs, French and Canadian fur traders, in the eighteenth century, and parts of the BWCAW had active logging into the early twentieth century. Other areas contained cabins and resorts that were only accessible by motorboats and small airplanes, up until federal wilderness protections in the 1960s banned motors and removed the resorts.[35] Ecofeminists and environmental justice scholars have troubled dominant ideas about wilderness and nature for neglecting perspectives that situate nonhuman nature in people's everyday lives.[36] Getting away from civilization to the backwoods is a distinctly white and upper-class desire, while for African Americans and other people of color, being in remote places may stir feelings of fear and anxiety that are shaped by histories of racial violence and segregation.[37]

Is All Mining the Same?

The political-economic and symbolic power of mining means that all groups frame their positions in relation to existing iron mines. Some struggles, then, center on whether new copper-nickel and legacy iron mining are *basically the same* or *fundamentally different*. Environmental groups assert that copper-nickel mining is distinct from—and more dangerous than—existing iron mines, and most are careful to avoid direct critiques of iron mining. Pro-mining groups argue that copper-nickel mining is not fundamentally different or riskier than the iron mining that has defined the area for well over a century.

The environmentalists have scientific evidence on their side here, although that is not to say that some do not exaggerate and overgeneralize the risks. Copper-nickel mines are riskier than iron mines. In fact, such nonferrous hardrock mining is one of the largest sources of Superfund sites in the US—so designated based on their extensive environmental damage and cleanup costs.[38] To call attention to these risks, environmental groups strategically refer to copper-nickel mining as "sulfide mining." This emphasizes how acid mine drainage poses threats to nearby waterways. Jennifer, who is in her fifties, explained that the organization she works for got involved in the fights over PolyMet on this basis: "And partially it's—this type of mining [copper-nickel] has never been done intentionally in Minnesota. It has such a bad track record both environmentally and financially in other states. It was—for those who were sort of even paying attention at all, there was a recognition that this is different than taconite and this is something we ought to really be more cautious about." Later, Jennifer added, "We are not anti-taconite [iron mining], and we are not anti-sulfide mining. But we do treat them differently because we think that the history of sulfide mining is such that it is quite a riskier proposition." Riskier, with a "bad track record," and out of place in Minnesota—to her, copper-nickel mining is a bridge too far. Without challenging the culturally and politically powerful iron industry, she presents her organization's position as reasonable, pro-development, and informed by science.

Most of the environmental organizations involved with copper-nickel mining are mainstream groups focused on policy, law, and public education. They, too, publicly state that they are *not* anti-mining—they do not want to shut down existing iron mines or disparage the mining legacy. Most groups working against the PolyMet project say, for instance, that they are only demanding that mining companies prove they can meet environmental regulations and pay for any cleanup that becomes necessary (a potentially spurious claim, since it may be technically or financially impossible for companies to meet these standards). The CSBW specifies that it is not anti-mining, only opposed to mining in a particular place (the BWCAW and its watershed), again attempting not to alienate locals who are proud of the area's iron mining history and to counter conservative rhetoric about environmentalists being extremists who are anti-development and anti-progress.

A few smaller, grassroots groups take a stronger position, opposing copper-nickel mining outright. It is not about individual projects for these groups but wholesale opposition to multinational corporations' profit-seeking on public lands and to copper-nickel mining, which they claim cannot be done safely in Minnesota. A few environmental groups are willing to, if cautiously, critique iron mining, underscoring demands for state agencies to uphold existing environmental regulations. MCEA and WaterLegacy have filed lawsuits to this effect, charging that state agencies have failed to enforce pollution standards, particularly the sulfate standard (a unique state regulation created primarily to protect wild rice), under political pressure from the iron-mining industry.[39] WaterLegacy has also worked with Ojibwe tribes to uphold and strengthen the sulfate rule in order to protect wild rice, particularly from iron mines that emit sulfates.

Pro-mining groups argue that this is all a façade. In their view, all environmentalists are anti-mining, and any attack on copper-nickel mining is an attack on Iron Rangers' collective history. "Nothing short of no mining in Minnesota would satisfy these anti-mining groups," reads a public statement from a white, male industry leader.[40] Like others who framed their opponents as ideologues out to stop mining and as looking down on people who rely on mining to make a living, Max described environmental organizations as "groups that would just as soon shut down all mining, including iron ore. . . . It's kind of a nondiscriminatory opposition to overall mining." Max, a leader of a mining-industry group, argues that environmentalists are coming to get iron mining and destroy the Iron Range way of life.

Given the weakness of environmental regulations, it is highly unlikely that environmental groups—or *any* group—truly could shut down the operating iron mines. However, on the Iron Range, there is some historical precedent giving resonance to these claims. In 1974, a federal judge made a landmark environmental law decision, ordering Reserve Mining to shut its taconite plant and build a new waste-storage facility to prevent further pollution of Lake Superior.[41] An appeals court partially reversed the decision, allowing Reserve Mining to reopen within a few days, though it upheld the requirement that the company build a new waste facility.[42] Nearly fifty years later, my interviews and casual conversations turned up numerous comments on the impacts of that temporary closure, and it was clear that memories about the bitter fights over Reserve Mining remain fresh. Today, the facility is owned and operated by Cleveland Cliffs, only a few miles from its onetime company town, Babbitt, and from the proposed PolyMet mine site.

Mine supporters also reject opponents' separation of nonferrous and ferrous mining, calling it mere rhetorical difference. They argue that copper-nickel mining uses the same basic processes as iron mining, that it is being proposed for the same place with essentially the same rocks that have been mined for generations, and that it can be done safely with a few additional environmental protections. Indeed, residents' lived experiences with relatively benign iron mining contradict environmentalists' claims of devastation, contributing to their sense that new copper-nickel mines are not the environmental threat that opponents assert. In an op-ed for a local newspaper, a state legislator wrote, "After more than 125 years of iron ore mining on the Range, one would have to ask, 'What don't we know about mining that hasn't been learned in the last 125 years?'"[43] This deploys a commonsense logic yet ignores real differences in the chemical compositions of and geological formations that contain iron and copper ores (and that carry different pollution risks). Recall the *Ely Echo*'s editorial in favor of the Twin Metals project, quoted earlier, and its sarcastic framing: after 130 years of mining, the author writes triumphantly, "by some miracle you can drink the water and eat the fish. . . . Imagine that."[44]

Dominant collective memories that remember iron mining as *clean* are examples of what science journalist and professor Deborah Rudacille calls "toxic nostalgia." In this variant, communities paradoxically long for a return to an industrial past, though the facilities demonstrably poisoned workers, created public health problems, and contaminated surrounding ecosystems.[45] Toxic, like smokestack, nostalgia glosses over past environmental problems from iron mining and lends trust to the idea that new mining projects will be clean job-creation hubs. And it overlooks the documented hazards created by copper-nickel mining, including extensive global pollution and water contamination tied to nonferrous hardrock mining.[46]

To be clear, northern Minnesota's waters are already polluted. The St. Louis River, downstream from the iron mines, was placed on American Rivers' most-endangered list in 2015.[47] Researchers find that the areas of northern Minnesota with lower water quality are also more likely to be near mining, while the areas with cleaner water tend to have less mining and industrial activity nearby.[48] Extracting iron releases atmospheric mercury and sulfates, which damage wild rice habitat and spur mercury's toxic methylation.[49] Chemicals, dust, and other cast-offs create occupational and public health hazards, including the release of hazardous asbestiform fibers into the air and water. Minnesota's Department of Health has documented elevated rates of mesothelioma, a rare respiratory cancer associated with asbestos, in this region and among former mine workers.[50] A longitudinal study of mine workers' health reports higher than expected rates of cardiovascular disease and lung cancer.[51]

Notably, all this pollution is essentially invisible. Iron Range residents' experience with visibly clean lakes, of catching and eating fish without experiencing noticeable, direct health problems, provides powerful experiential knowledge. Their everyday interactions affirming the anecdotal safety of mining can be more powerful than abstract scientific evidence, especially when those experiences align with dominant ideologies about mining as a way of life and corporate public relations. Recognizing that mining has damaged and will damage the environment means forcing people to recognize the dissonance between their conflicting mining and outdoor-recreation identities. It disrupts their idyllic memories of the good old days in ways that are uncomfortable. Instead, many return to their own, firsthand understandings that the risks are low and the potential rewards are high.

Contested Assessments of the Future

How people perceive the risks and benefits of proposed industries depends on how they remember the history of an industry.[52] Pro-mining groups remember iron mining as being clean. Environmental groups remember the opposite, that it was not environmentally safe and that companies and regulators will do little to address future pollution threats. For the industry to convince locals to support its copper-nickel proposals, optimistic corporate forecasts of mineral abundance, job creation, revenue, and clean mining must be backed by individuals' sense that these claims are credible.[53] When the companies' rhetoric fits well with collective memories, this is more likely.

Even so, supporters do not just blindly trust copper-nickel-mining companies to protect the environment. Alex, a union staff member, told me that he has many concerns when it comes to PolyMet and Twin Metals. He wants to see strong evidence that the mines can be operated and closed safely. Hank, a retired miner who now works in real estate in Ely, likewise supports *exploration* for copper-nickel mining, provided that it follow all regulations. If the companies prove that mining can be done safely, he thinks the projects should move forward: "I don't want to be blind here. Growing up here, I know what we have, and I don't want anything to happen, like polluting the area." He continued, "This mining stuff, yeah, there's pros and cons. There's always going to be pollution. I don't care how careful you are. I don't want to see anything happen to us, to anybody." For Hank, granting the permits should hinge on whether mining companies can protect the place he cares about. Similarly, Tony, a union organizer, and his father, a retired miner in his late seventies, voiced support for the copper-nickel mines but attenuated that support with serious concerns based in what they saw as already-lax adherence to mining regulations and corporations prioritizing profits over the environment and public health.

Other residents were warier. Going on weekly guided nature walks around Ely, I got to know some of the regulars. When one of the other regulars—a woman in her sixties—heard that I was studying copper-nickel mining, she stopped to talk with me at the end of the hike. She was born in Ely, comes from a mining family, still lives nearby, and has friends who are pro-mining and support Twin Metals. Yet she is skeptical. She thinks the new mines are riskier than iron mines and does not trust company's safety claims that they will not pollute the area where people love to hunt and fish.

People involved with environmental and conservation organizations expectedly expressed even greater distrust in predictions from companies or regulators. Few of them shared the smokestack nostalgia I heard from longtime and working-class Iron Range residents. Instead, they remembered a legacy of environmental pollution, land degradation, and economic instability. Linda, a staff member at an environmental group, said bluntly, "the State of Minnesota has done an absolutely atrocious job of regulating the pollution" from taconite mines, and "we believe [those] are less toxic than copper-nickel mines." Another seasoned environmentalist and organization staff member, Amanda, lives in Duluth. She questioned PolyMet's claims about safety by connecting the future risks of copper-nickel mining to the industry's long history of pollution across the world and to the long timeline of environmental pollutants:

> I think that the number-one thing is that the pollution from [copper-nickel mines] lasts so long, so many years, hundreds, thousands of years into the future. There are still mines from the Roman Empire that are polluting water in Europe. At PolyMet, while they're going to have a water-treatment plant that is going to treat the polluted discharge from the mine pits, we have no idea what's going to happen in the future as far as our social and economic and regulatory systems. The idea that what we've got now is going to continue for a thousand years with no breaks . . . The experience in the past is that mining companies always underpredict what the impacts on water quality are going to be.

In her assessment, companies often underestimate future contamination—and how far into the future that contamination will persist.

In public messaging, opposition groups often turn to the time horizons of pollution. Wastewater and runoff from mines, they note, will need to be stored in perpetuity; the potential that these waste materials will generate acids and heavy metals cannot be eliminated. Five hundred years of pollution, a number taken from PolyMet's calculations in its environmental impact statement, is an oft-cited figure, used to emphasize that the risks will far outlast any single company. Gary, the owner of an outdoor-recreation company and leader in the CSBW, talked about the symbolic power of that number: "When you look at the PolyMet EIS, they talk about 'five hundred years of treatment'—five hundred years, no big deal. We as humans have a hard time understanding geologic time. We can't even understand five hundred years. That goes right over everybody's heads. Five hundred years. . . . This [the US] has been a republic for, what, two hundred fifty years or something?" For critics, five hundred years of pollution risks handily outweigh the potential for twenty years of lucrative mining operations (not to mention the effects of another boom-and-bust cycle).

Both sides of the copper-nickel mining conflict assert moral claims about fighting for future generations and leaving behind a better world. Yet they disagree about what should be preserved and restored. When I asked Bill, a recreation guide and activist with the CSBW in his late thirties, about his perceptions of mine supporters, he reflected, "I think everybody wants the best. You know, I don't think anyone has ill intentions. Everyone just has a different idea of what they think is going to be best for our community and for the region. I think there is just disagreement over what we want the future to look like and, also, how likely it is that there would be significant pollution or negative effects from the mine."

For supporters, new mining would bring economic prosperity that could keep rural mining communities alive. They see an ethical obligation to promote mining so that their children and grandchildren, as the retired miner Randy suggested, will continue to live in the region and achieve the "good life." Marty, the retired Ely schoolteacher, was more certain: "I really think the only future that the Iron Range has is going to be in mining, without a doubt. That has been our lives, been our life throughout. I think it's going to be in the future." I find that these sorts of desires to provide for the next generation contributes to trusting corporate forecasts of job creation.

Emil Ramirez, director of the United Steelworkers (USW) District 11, wrote in an op-ed for the *Duluth News Tribune*, "At a time when too many families live with employment insecurity, we cannot allow this rare opportunity to create family-supporting, community-sustaining jobs slip away. With a viable business plan, a skilled workforce, and a market that has found its footing, we have confidence in NorthMet [the name of PolyMet's mine project] and sincerely believe in the project's ability to deliver on its promise of a more prosperous future in an environmentally responsible manner."[54] Again, we see the framing of a new mine project as a *necessary* solution for the region's problems, a way to restore the community's health and vibrancy that is likely to pose few environmental risks.

The promise of technological advancements is another way that mine supporters claim the copper-nickel mines will be safe. Trust in technology reflects an ecomodernist masculinity in which engineering and industrial progress are seen as the path to environmental sustainability. That this argument has historical precedent in the Iron Range gives additional legitimacy to the companies' predictions. For example, a new method for processing low-grade iron ore (taconite) provided a technological fix in the 1950s that extended the life of the region's iron-mining industry, bringing jobs and revenue in a moment when the high-grade iron-ore reserves had been depleted.[55] Using a new processing technique designed by a researcher at the University of Minnesota, Edward W. Davis, lower-grade taconite could be converted into iron pellets for use in steel foundries.[56] The first of these taconite plants was the Reserve Mining Company project in Babbitt, but it was soon followed by other companies and new company towns like Hoyt Lakes. The taconite boom lasted through the early 1970s, and it is this type of mining that continues at the operating mines in the region.[57]

Older Iron Range residents are from a generation that started their careers in the taconite mines or remembered their fathers going to work in these facilities. And their memories give the PolyMet plans particular symbolic resonance; these call for constructing the new mine site near Babbitt and repurposing the old Erie/LTV Mining taconite-processing facility in Hoyt Lakes. In other words, PolyMet claims that it can transform the birthplace of taconite into the birthplace of copper-nickel mining. Longtime residents have seen it happen before, so why would they not be inclined to believe it could happen again?

Further, Iron Rangers' hopeful support for extractive development is about revitalizing a sense of community and pride. Mining supporters, like those quoted earlier, expressed emotional desires about a return to lively towns with bright futures. Tim, the Hoyt Lakes retiree, spoke of this directly during our conversation on his back patio: "[PolyMet] would generate more of an upbeat atmosphere, of course, and there'd be new people coming in that wanted maybe a different business in town. There'd be more money flowing for sure. We're basically now—we are either on welfare or retired."

One thing my respondents seem to overlook is that mine closures alone are not the reason for the lack of good jobs. Iron mines, after all, are still operating here. But automation and mechanization—processes that also impact copper-nickel mining—reduced the amount of labor needed to mine iron in the 1930s and the 1960s, and surely they will continue to do so into the future. The copper-nickel-mining companies also plan to mine low-grade, deposits which require low operation costs to be profitable; they will be under enormous pressure to limit labor expenses. The jobs they do offer will require high-skilled and technical laborers, an indication that they may bring in outside workers rather than hire extensively from the local labor pool. And, as noted, some of the initial permit applications are for only twenty years of operation. To the extent that locals will see a job boon, it may only last through the initial construction of the copper-nickel-mining facilities. This is where critics return to the troubling boom-and-bust cycles of extractive development.

Still, in an area plagued by social and economic challenges, some jobs and even a short-lived revival are better than none. Alternative economic development is a challenge in the isolated and rural regions developed around natural resources; today, the company towns left behind are often isolated places with limited infrastructure to support incoming industries. Few viable options are on offer for reviving the Iron Range economy, and a history of failed development and economic diversification attempts redouble local skepticism about the efficacy of transitioning away from mining. In one painful episode, policy makers leveraged public funds and tax incentives to attract solar-panel factories, which employed only a few workers and mostly failed. Only a single factory remains open.[58] Still, some local leaders I spoke with were more circumspect in their support of copper-nickel mining and did not see the industry as a panacea for the region's woes. I chatted with an Ely city council member—the only woman on the council at the time—who sees herself as a bridge builder. She thinks that copper-nickel mining should go forward if it passes regulatory scrutiny but is not waiting around for the projects to save the day. Thus, she is active in revitalizing Ely's downtown, fostering local arts and theater, and developing broadband internet.

Opponents of Twin Metals and PolyMet think the region's future will require more creative thinking, beyond the focus on a romanticized past, and that more mining would hamper alternatives. When I asked Elliot, a young CSBW staff member in Ely, about the social dynamics in town, he said that he thinks the mining supporters are, to some degree, stuck in the past: "I think that there's more of people looking in the rearview mirror. Like, 'Mining is the only thing we need, and we just got to do that.' There's the other group, which is like, 'No, we can do other stuff'—trying to figure out a different future for the town."

At times, critiques of local mining supporters could be classist and patronizing. During one of the regular volunteer-led nature walks I went on, a fellow hiker, who lives in Florida and owns a lake cabin near Ely, lamented that some of the locals are stuck in the past and only want more mining but could not see the risks and downsides. He is personally worried that industrialization and pollution from mining could drive down the value of his lakefront property.

Neither messaging or policy proposals from environmental groups have emphasized just transitions that would move the region toward a socioenvironmentally sustainable economy while providing decent and meaningful jobs for Iron Rangers. They have not articulated a clear alternative vision that resonates with Iron Rangers' collective memories, hopes, and material concerns. They speak of tourism and recreation as economic drivers, though these do not necessarily provide good jobs or solutions for the majority of Iron Rangers, who do not live adjacent to the popular BWCAW or have the requisite skills or interests. Nor does working as a retail clerk, a waiter, or a guide at an outfitting company provide culturally and socially meaningful forms of work, especially for men who desire industrial and physical labor. Most recreation and hospitality jobs do not provide careers with decent wages, benefits, and consistent hours—like the cherished iron-mining jobs. Yes, expecting environmental groups to come up with solutions to major economic-development challenges may be asking too much. The groups are small organizations with limited capacity, and they focus their limited resources on political and legal efforts to challenge powerful, deep-pocketed industries. Still, more could be done to frame the issue around just transitions for mining communities and workers, to present a hopeful vision for the future that holds water with workers and rural residents.

Conclusion

Conflicts over the use of natural resources and environmental conservation are animated by emotional meanings attached to the past and visions for the future. Copper-nickel mining's support from working-class and rural residents and opposition from largely urban, suburban, and middle-class environmentalists are both driven by nostalgia, fears of loss, and hopes toward securing the good life for future generations. Yet what people fear losing and what they want to restore differs depending on their timescapes, varying across class, gender, race, and place.

My exploration of the way these different notions of time inform environmental politics and activism in this region has offered three important conclusions. First, environmental issues are understood and contested through emotional meanings of the past and future, not just economic interests or assessments of scientific and technical data. Temporality and emotion are key dynamics for how social movements, politicians, and corporations work to mobilize support and construct legitimacy. Appeals to collective memories and nostalgia are effective framing strategies that create personal and emotional connections to often-technical issues about regulatory decision-making, mine engineering plans, and water-quality modeling.

Second, while I argue that job creation alone does not explain rural, working-class support for hazardous industries, political-economic conditions still shape the power of nostalgia and hope to sustain the legitimacy of extractive capitalism. Volatile extractive economies produce idyllic memories of boom times and anxieties about painful memories of busts.[59] In rural mining regions that are experiencing deindustrialization and disinvestment, smokestack nostalgia appeals. It fits with memories of a bygone era of prosperity based on masculine industrial jobs, contrasted with current-day economic struggles and fears about losing a sense of community. Smokestack nostalgia allows for an alluring, hopeful vision of the future that is tangible and reaffirms collective identities of place, masculinity, and class.

Third, nostalgia is not inherently reactionary or progressive. Appeals to nostalgia are used by different political interests, including environmental movements and anti-environmental and right-wing movements. Nostalgia is a complex emotion that can be directed toward imagining more just futures just as easily as it can be mobilized to defend oppressive socioenvironmental relations.[60] The desire to restore a golden era—often based on patriarchy, white supremacy, and exploitation of labor and the environment—can mobilize a reactionary defense of place that supports extractive capitalism and fosters resentment toward outsiders (often understood as government, urban elites, immigrants, and environmentalists). Yet this same nostalgia can be mobilized to valorize struggles against mine bosses and affirm worker and community solidarity in the face of economic and political challenges. Nostalgia can *also* energize a progressive defense of place that resists expanded extractivism and advocates for alternative development and democratic decision-making about land and resource use. Thus, mining companies encounter resistance when they pursue development in places where people have competing collective memories linked to outdoor recreation and environmental conservation.

All forms of nostalgia gloss over the problematic aspects of history. Smokestack nostalgia valorizes an industry associated with environmental degradation, worker exploitation, and oppressive gender relations.[61] Wilderness nostalgia overlooks how the area that is now the BWCAW is not simply an untrammeled landscape but a site shaped by industrial and human activity for millennia. It erases the legacy of Indigenous displacement, presuming a particular white, middle-class way of relating to nonhuman nature and "doing" outdoor recreation that may not resonate or be accessible for local Indigenous people, rural white people, working-class people, or people of color.

5

Extractive Populism

Defending the Iron Range Way of Life

On a summer afternoon in 2017, I met Tom, a retired miner and former union member, at his house in Ely, a northern Minnesota town that abuts the Boundary Waters. He was talking with a neighbor and tinkering with a vintage car as I pulled up in my Toyota Prius. I was barely parked before the men launched into a series of jokes about my car, the stereotypical transport of urban environmentalists (made by a foreign company, to boot). "Don't they give tickets for parking a Prius in Ely?" Then Tom announced his intention to set me straight: I had probably talked to some of the environmentalists in town, but he was going to tell me the real story.

Tom's initial wariness gave way as he learned that my grandfather had grown up in nearby Hibbing—my Finnish surname had roots up here. For an hour or so, he shared stories about his life and his family, especially how they made a living in logging and mining for several generations. Then Tom said that I should come see his family's land and the lakeside log cabin his father had built a few miles outside of town.

Driving out of town along a tree-lined two-lane highway in his 1970s Chevy Camaro, Tom slammed on the accelerator and gave me a masculine display of the car's power. Once we slowed down, we started talking politics. Tom described himself as an "old-fashioned Democrat," pro-life and pro-gun, and told me that he had been involved with the DFL his entire life. Now, he remarked, it seemed that the Democratic Party was no longer for "us." Party leadership in the Twin Cities had drifted away from working people's issues like jobs and mining. With a twinkle, Tom said he figured I would be surprised that he actually caucused for Bernie Sanders, a self-declared socialist, in the 2016 Democratic primary. By the election, the party's candidate was Hillary Clinton—whom Tom saw as both deceitful and a third-term proxy for Bill Clinton, whose trade policies had hurt the working class. And so, the lifelong DFL activist smiled and said, "It was a good thing the ballot box was private."

How did a union member and longtime Democratic activist come to support, at least tacitly, Donald Trump, a right-wing politician and wealthy businessman from New York City? How was this switch related to conflicts over Minnesota's proposed copper-nickel mines? And how does right-wing populism come to be seen as protecting rural working-class ways of life, despite its pro-business and anti-worker stances?

The rightward swing of rural, white, and working-class voters highlighted by the 2016 election sparked renewed interested in rural and postindustrial places in the Midwest and Northeast. Trump won in Iron Range precincts that went for Barack Obama four years prior, that had not voted for a Republican presidential candidate since the 1930s—and this dynamic played out well beyond northeastern Minnesota, spilling into other traditional Democratic strongholds like Wisconsin, Ohio, and Pennsylvania. In 2020, Trump again won the Eighth Congressional District, which encompasses the Iron Range, although Democrat Joe Biden did improve on Hillary Clinton's showing in 2016 and won the vote in some Iron Range cities. This rightward shift has been met with an outpouring of commentary, press coverage, and scholarship about the white working class and why they support conservative politicians. The usual explanations included racism, xenophobia, and the impacts of economic dislocation.[1]

I contend that, amid a national surge in right-wing populism mobilized by the Tea Party movement and then Trump and his allies, conservative politicians have successfully appealed to the cultural and ideological meanings of mining, rural places, masculinity, and class in a discourse of *extractive populism*. In northern Minnesota, the conflict over copper-nickel mines is inextricable from this rightward political shift. It has opened schisms in the Democratic coalition, amplifying rural-urban divides (at least voters' perceptions of their importance) and positioning job creation and environmental conservation as oppositional goals. Mine supporters present copper-nickel mining as a tangible way to defend the region's rural moral economy against threats and outsiders like urban elite environmentalists and federal bureaucrats, to renew a prosperous mining heritage based in stable and masculine industrial jobs, and to promote national security by securing domestic sources of metals. The cultural and social aspects of class and masculinity are mobilized in sowing rural-versus-urban divisions and framing corporations as the champions of male working-class livelihoods and lifestyles tied to extractive industries. This rhetoric resonated with Trump's "Make America Great Again" tagline and his populist appeals to the "people," like claims about putting coal miners back to work.[2] In contrast, environmental populists yearn for clean air and water for future generations and public lands open for all Americans to enjoy, rather than being reserved for private profit-making.

Political Splits over Copper-Nickel Mining

Conflicts over the copper-nickel-mining projects are driving a wedge into the DFL by exacerbating divisions between the party's rural and urban and labor and environmental wings. The complex politics of mining were summed up by a house I drove by ten miles outside of Ely, where a "Bernie for President" (referring to Bernie Sanders, the democratic-socialist from Vermont running in the 2016 Democratic presidential primary) sign sat in the front lawn alongside a "We Support Mining" sign. Tony, a union organizer and political activist in northeastern Minnesota, painted the picture this way: "We don't have a DFL up on the Range. We practice our own. . . . We call ourselves 'DFL,' but it's our own version of it. They're [the Iron Range] separating themselves completely from that Duluth bunch that's trying to take over and that Twin Cities bunch, but at the same time, there's part of the Duluth bunch that is still pro-labor and still pro-mining, so there's all kinds of little factions and camps going on."

Broadly, Iron Range DFL politicians strongly support the copper-nickel-mining projects, while their Twin Cities– and Duluth-based colleagues are critical. Statewide politicians, like the governor and both US senators, have tried to navigate a balanced position by supporting PolyMet but not Twin Metals, by advocating for rigorous scientific review but not outright opposition to the approval of permits. For example, Governor Mark Dayton (who served from 2011 to 2019) publicly supported the PolyMet project if it met all permit requirements but expressed doubt about the Twin Metals project and mining within the watershed of the BWCAW.[3] Rather than striking balance and cultivating support, Dayton's stance created anger among pro-mining groups, including some Democrats, and resulted in the Ely-based group Up North Jobs bringing a lawsuit against the governor. At the same time, Dayton was criticized by environmentalists for his support of PolyMet.

The DFL's within-party tensions were on display when the environmental caucus at the 2016 party convention introduced Resolution 54, a proposal that would have made the party's platform opposed to copper-nickel mining (which they called "sulfide ore mining"). The resolution was defeated after vocal opposition, but the struggle laid bare the distrust and animosity building within the party. The *Mesabi Daily News* speculated the Resolution 54 vote "could create a deep rift between Range DFLers and the party as a whole, jeopardizing a historically close-knit allegiance with the region."[4]

Support for copper-nickel mining generated political realignments as Iron Range DFLers worked with Republicans in Minnesota and beyond to promote mining. The former congressman Rick Nolan is a case in point: he had supported copper-nickel-mining projects, even introducing and sponsoring federal legislation to advance the PolyMet and Twin Metals proposals, and he opposed state and federal actions to deny mineral leases near the BWCAW or add additional environmental reviews. Nolan and Minnesota's Sixth District Republican congressman Tom Emmer worked together to create an amendment defunding a US Forest Service environmental impact study of copper-nickel mining in the BWCAW watershed.[5] Nolan's "yes" vote on another Emmer-penned bill, known as Minnesota's Economic Rights (MINER) Act, in 2017 attracted particular attention. The MINER Act would have renewed federal mineral leases denied to Twin Metals under the Obama administration, ended the environmental review of mining in the BWCAW watershed, and eliminated the ability of federal agencies to withdraw mineral leases in the future.[6] Its potential to upend federal land and mineral policies attracted the attention of Republicans in western states, who wanted to weaken federal control of land and environmental protections. However, most Minnesota Democrats, particularly representatives covering the Twin Cities, opposed the bill, as did one Republican congressman, Erik Paulsen from a district near Minneapolis. Thus, Republicans and Democrats aligned on both sides of the issue—something particularly rare in this period of rancorous partisan divides.

Republicans have sought to lock up the votes of working-class and rural whites since at least the 1960s. Right-wing populist groups and political leaders, claiming to stand up for this silent majority, have come to ascribe blame for their economic and social woes on government bureaucrats, immigrants, people of color, and liberal urban elites.[7] But while mining, industrial, and rural regions such as Appalachia and the Rust Belt responded, with voters shifting to the right in the 1980s and more so in the 2010s, Minnesota's Iron Range remained a holdout.[8] The postwar liberal alliance of labor, farmers, and urban progressives in the Democratic Party (known as the DFL in Minnesota) held, however tenuously.

The historian Jeffrey T. Manuel argues that the Iron Range's conservative reticence owes to a set of relatively successful efforts to address deindustrialization and maintain its mining industry.[9] Unions including the United Steelworkers remained strong throughout the 1980s, and adept and pragmatic political leaders, like former US senator Paul Wellstone, embodied a form of progressive populism that spoke to labor concerns and maintained the alignment of rural and urban voters. However, continued industrial decline, demographic changes, the rise of new politicians and new politics, and cultural shifts have served to destabilize the liberal coalition in Minnesota.

Until Trump, no Republican presidential candidate had won the Iron Range since Herbert Hoover in 1928.[10] Statewide, Hillary Clinton edged out Trump in 2016 (46.4 percent to 44.9 percent), but Trump carried much of northeastern Minnesota—in some Iron Range precincts, by as much as 15 percent. Some of the region's largest cities, including Hibbing and Virginia, went decisively for Obama in 2012, then chose Trump four years later.[11] The rightward pull filtered down the ballot, turning the US congressional race for Minnesota's Eighth District—long a DFL bastion—into one of the country's most hotly contested and expensive races. In 2016, the DFL incumbent, Rick Nolan, barely held onto his seat, eking out a win by around two thousand votes, partially by taking an adamantly pro-mining position.[12] In 2018, however, Nolan did not run, and Republican Pete Stauber took the seat in a fairly large victory, beating the DFL candidate, Joe Radinovich, 50.7 percent to 45.2 percent.

Tom, in Ely, was not alone in supporting Bernie Sanders, who won Minnesota's statewide 2016 Democratic primary election by twenty-three

TABLE 5.1. Federal Voting Results in the Minnesota Iron Range, 2012 and 2016

Precinct	US Congress (Eighth District)		US presidential election							
	2012	2016	2012				2016			
	Nolan (D)	Nolan (D)	Obama (D)	Romney (R)	Stein (Green)	Johnson (Libertarian)	Clinton (D)	Trump (R)	Stein (Green)	Johnson (Libertarian)
6A	64.48 percent	59.25 percent	62.96 percent	34.44 percent	0.43 percent	1.13 percent	44.23 percent	47.36 percent	1.25 percent	3.47 percent
6B	58.03 percent	56.01 percent	61.62 percent	35.78 percent	0.48 percent	1.18 percent	44.62 percent	47.31 percent	1.27 percent	3.50 percent
3A	56.18 percent	54.93 percent	55.06 percent	42.16 percent	0.45 percent	1.27 percent	42.72 percent	49.17 percent	1.38 percent	3.13 percent

percentage points (in the Eighth Congressional District, Sanders took 65 percent).[13] By the 2016 general election, voters continued to show a preference for anti-establishment candidates: the Green Party candidate, Jill Stein, and the Libertarian candidate, Gary Johnson, each earned more votes than they had in 2012 (see table 5.1). That Trump carried the region in 2016 and 2020 (though he lost the state both times) underscores voters' rising sense that neither of the traditional parties speaks for their interests.

Extractive Populism in the Iron Range

I use the term *extractive populism*, building on the geographer Matthew Huber's concept of "energy populism" related to the dominance of oil in US political-economy and culture, to describe the symbolic, cultural, and ideological power of mining, the strategies used to legitimize extractive industries, and the role of resource extraction in right-wing populist movements and rural mobilization.[14] In the current case, supporters of new copper-nickel mines in Minnesota frame the projects as a way for rural Iron Rangers to reclaim power from outsiders and elites, provide the jobs and materials necessary for the "good life," restore a mining heritage, and promote national security through resource independence. Extractive populism is intertwined with hegemonic masculinity, seen in appeals to restore a threatened masculinity and defend the nation—indicative of the way the cultural, social, and emotional meanings of fossil fuels and extractive industries are mobilized to defend white patriarchy.[15] Through extractive populism, deregulation and opening up public lands for development by private corporations are positioned as moves promoting the interests of *the people*.[16] Yet not all Iron Rangers have bought into this discourse, and I met many people who were ambivalent about copper-nickel mining and did not long for a return to the past—they were actively creating other futures through small businesses, arts and entertainment, and education. In this chapter, I focus on those who are ardent mining supporters and how politicians and other corporate and civic leaders frame copper-nickel mining.

Extractive populism implicitly appeals to idealized white, working-class, masculine, and rural ways of life, based in physically challenging mining jobs with family-supporting wages, and a sense of threat to the economic and moral status of dominant white masculinity. While issues of race were largely silent among the mostly white people I met, race and racism were still important forces. As race scholars show, contemporary forms of racism often operate by silencing direct discussion of race with color-blind rhetoric, presumptions of dominant whiteness, and the coded language of dog-whistle politics.[17] We see this in right-wing populist appeals to defend the "people," which is based on a white imaginary alongside racialized fears about cities and immigrants.[18]

As I explored in chapter 4, Iron Range towns are now dominated by a nostalgic populist narrative about defending their way of life. Developing copper-nickel mines is presented as a way to protect a rural moral economy and unearth an idealized past—one white pro-mining activist described his vision for the region as going "back to what we used to be." This moral economy was based around the male breadwinner who did physically tough and dangerous work in the mines to provide for his family and community. Like residents of other rural US regions, Iron Rangers develop their views on political and social issues on the basis of a perception of collective interests, not solely individual, and a desire to protect their community's sense of moral standing against a myriad of perceived threats, from deindustrialization to changing cultural norms.[19]

In my conversation with Chris, a midfifties white Elyite, he also subtly referenced the nostalgic tone of Trumpian "Make America Great Again" politics: "When I was growing up, everybody's parents, or dad at least, worked there [the iron mine]. Women didn't work really. Everybody had a stay-at-home mom. But at that point in time, those were good union jobs. So everybody was making good money. It was a middle-class town. We didn't have any extreme poverty, and we didn't have any extreme wealth. . . . Growing up like that, you never wanted for anything." For Chris, the "good life" at the heart of the region's moral economy involved a tacit agreement: male workers would put in long, demanding hours in the mines, for which their union ensured they got decent wages and benefits that allowed them to support their families and create stable communities.

This vision of a moral economy based around decent jobs for white men in exchange for supporting mining corporations, which profit from extracting value from the land, has now been disrupted. Automation, resource depletion, and outsourcing have meant the loss of mining jobs and economic stability. They have also threatened masculinity, as men lose out on high-paying industrial jobs; the only growth areas are in the stereotypically feminine industries of health care, service, and tourism. Right-wing populist messages recognize these threats and insecurities, blame them on outsider environmentalists and government bureaucracy, and position copper-nickel mines as the solution to renew an idealized past.

In the summer of 2017, pro-mining groups organized a rally that they described as "for our way of life," before a public hearing on the PolyMet project. Social media messages touted the event as a fight for the future of the Range. Union leaders and pro-mining politicians spoke at the rally, carefully and consistently describing the region's way of life—inseparable from mining—as weathering a sustained attack. St. Louis County Commissioner Tom Rukavina (DFL), an iconic political figure in the region, said of environmentalists and urbanites, "They always want to 'save the lynx' and 'save the wolves.' The only thing they don't want to save is our way of life. We're proud of what we do!"

Rob, a pro-mining activist, found hope in messages like these, telling me that he thought Trump would help the working class. As a candidate, Rob said, Trump "was for the American people. He was for the American workers. . . . He wanted to bring business back to this country. Those are the things that your normal, everyday working guy wanted to hear instead of watching their jobs go overseas because of excessive taxes and restrictions." In this vision, putting men back to work and defending the US means expanding resource extraction, limiting imports, and cutting environmental regulations. Yet even many Trump supporters acknowledged that he alone could not open the copper-nickel mines and bring jobs to the region. Their votes signal that Trump's populist appeal was not only about potential material benefits but also his connection to Iron Rangers' emotions and worldviews. A vote for Trump was a vote for the renewal of moral economies tied to extractive industries and defense of rural, working-class, white identities.

Outsiders versus Insiders

Us-versus-them rhetoric appeals to Iron Rangers' sense of collective belonging and solidarity and a shared history of survival in a harsh, isolated climate. It promises stability in the face of economic struggles and sociopolitical change, and it is nothing new. Animosity toward outsiders has a long legacy in this region, where politicians and labor leaders have fostered collective identity and solidarity to be mobilized against outsiders and to protect regional interests.[20] In the early to mid-twentieth century, the collective identity was panethnic, uniting laborers whose collective efficacy staved off some of the worst abuses of absentee East Coast mine bosses.

Whether it is East Coast mine bosses or urban environmentalists or the federal government, Iron Rangers' anger at outsiders is rooted in the idea that "they" want to tell "us" how to live.[21] Today, the pejorative term that these workers once used for outside strikebreakers, "packsackers," is instead applied to environmentalists and newcomers who are drawn to the area for its outdoor recreation. The "us" is equated with "old Ely," the multigeneration residents whose families immigrated from Europe to work in mining and logging, and "them" with "new Ely," the retirees, young people, and teleworkers who have moved to the area and bought up houses and lake cabins near the BWCAW in recent decades. Iron Rangers often cite how many generations their family has lived in the region and worked in the mines. "Old Ely" roughly corresponded to the city limits, within which the median family income was $36,059 in 2015, 41.5 percent of adults (including retirees) were out of the workforce, and 48.4 percent of voters voted for Trump in the 2016 election. Outside Ely, in its surrounding townships, housing costs were higher, as were median incomes ($54,022 in nearby Morse Township and $62,500 in Fall Lake Township, where many of the "new Elyites" live) and the percentage of adults out of the workforce (60 percent), indicating more retirees.[22] There are also political differences. More people outside of Ely's town boundaries voted Democratic in the 2016 election.[23]

People relocating to the area for the wilderness and natural beauty creates anxiety for longtime residents, who see their sense of community and way of life in jeopardy. "What if the gastropubs serving microbrew IPAs and global fusion cuisine on Ely's main street replace the old-timers' bars, where cans of Grain Belt are paired with potato chips?" This process, what some scholars call "rural gentrification," is causing conflicts in many areas of the US, as people with the means to do so move to areas with outdoor amenities, like Montana and Colorado.[24] To Randy, the newcomers in Ely and its surroundings are "a little two-faced": "They're fine as long as they got theirs and nobody else can. But that's part of the people that are moving here. They are like my age, retired people, that have had good jobs, so they don't need a job [now]. So they're fine and dandy with nothing happening here. They don't see any need for the industry or anything like that." Old Ely, on the other hand, needs industrial revitalization and paths forward for those who are increasingly tempted to leave the Range to provide stability for their families. New residents with different cultural tastes, white-collar jobs, and no connection to mining, Randy seemed to say, are a threat to rural livelihoods and ways of life.

All these us-versus-them categories draw on stereotypes. People who have relocated to the area are not a uniform group. Many of the newcomers I met, including those who are active in environmental groups, are middle-class professionals like teachers, nurses, and public employees. They live in fairly modest houses. They do not fit with the caricature of jet-setting urbanites building lakeside vacation homes with little concern for local issues. Take Bob, whom I met going on nature walks. He is a retired middle-school science teacher from Illinois who spends his summers birding, boating, and fishing around his small cabin—it has running water but no electricity—on the Kawishiwi River. He is not active in environmental groups but is skeptical of copper-nickel mining and concerned about water pollution and disruptions to the serene and beautiful place. Other people I met own small businesses in town and are active in civic organizations, like the volunteer at a small local history museum in Ely who moved to town three years ago from Omaha, Nebraska, and took over the local electronics store with her husband. She has a background in accounting, which she draws on to help the museum and the local golf club—popular with old-timers—manage their finances. Despite living in town and being active in the community, she feels like some people treat her as an outsider and do not like tourists, even though tourism is why Ely is faring better than other Iron Range towns are.

I learned that the class differences between new and old Elyites, between mining critics and supporters, are less about *wealth* than about the cultural and social dynamics of class and rural-versus-urban divisions. A retired iron miner in Ely might have a larger pension and heftier savings than a retired teacher who moved to the area to enjoy the wilderness. But the newer residents tend to have higher levels of formal education and different cultural tastes than longtime residents do—what the social theorist Pierre Bourdieu describes as social and cultural capital that influence people's status and social networks.[25] The groups differ with regard to the businesses they frequent, groups they participate in, and forms of recreation they enjoy. New Elyites might go to the contemporary restaurant with large glass windows and a reclaimed-wood bar serving locally sourced ingredients, shop at the town's fledgling natural foods store, or establish new groups like the Ely Folk School, which holds workshops on traditional crafts and folk music. People who identify as "old Ely," on the other hand, are skeptical toward businesses like the New Age wellness and healing center, which look like a sign of cultural change that is out of step with their community. They gather at legacy bars serving Grain Belt and whiskey and restaurants like the stalwart Ely Steakhouse serving burgers and T-bone steaks with dark-green carpets and wood paneling, and they join established groups including the Veterans of Foreign Wars (VFW) and antique car clubs.

To be sure, the groups are not entirely segregated. For example, a local summer opera production that features professional singers from around the world has been a decades-long tradition in towns across the Iron Range. Though opera does not fit with stereotypes about rural, working-class culture, the performance I attended in Ely was held in the ornate high school auditorium and attracted a large, diverse crowd of newcomer environmentalists right alongside longtime Ely residents and mine supporters. Performing in the auditorium of a rural high school was quite a shift for some of the singers, whose résumés include productions at world-class opera houses in Europe and major US cities. In another instance, I volunteered at the Northern Lake Arts Association Festival in Ely, which brought together a wide range of people to celebrate local artists and craftspeople. The lead organizers included recent transplants and longtime residents, and the art ranged from kitschy oil paintings of outdoor scenes to abstract mixed-media pieces. Near Hibbing, locals enjoy a long-running co-operative park that was started by radical Finnish immigrants (many of whom would have worked in the iron mines), and in Virginia, residents have welcomed the recent arrival of a co-operative grocery store.

In Ely, cultural class differences and conflicts have been most visible when they concern outdoor recreation. As discussed in chapter 1, divisions in the way people enjoy the outdoors have found cultural proxies in motorboats and canoes, oppositional stand-ins that have come to symbolize class and connection to place. The 1978 BWCAW Act banned motor vehicles in much of the area and reserved certain land for nonmotorized recreation. For many nearby residents, this action was seen as protecting middle-class and urbanite ways of experiencing nature. In other words, "old Ely" regards the limits placed on locals' ability to enjoy the place using motorized vehicles, from motorboats to snowmobiles, as the impositions of outside environmentalists and the federal government—both material and symbolic slights against their way of life.

Conflicts over copper-nickel mining are re-creating similar social rifts in Ely almost fifty years later. Karen, a middle-aged white woman who runs a small business in Ely and is involved in local conservation groups, recounted her return to Ely, after time away visiting family, with a shake of her head: "To come back and to see how much conflict and divide is going on in this community—more than the Trump situation, it's about this issue [copper-nickel mining]—and I think the current politics have kind of helped widen or elevated, I guess, exacerbate that divide." She felt alarmed by the rising tensions in her daily interactions, driven by conflicts over mining and national politics, as chats at the grocery store led to accusations that she was "anti-mining."

The 2017 Fourth of July parade in Ely drew several thousand people to downtown. Community groups like the Rotary Club, high school sports teams, and veterans' groups made floats and threw candy to kids. The owners of the local grocery store Zup's (named after the Slovenian-immigrant Zupancich family) wore clown costumes as they gave out boxes of Stove Top stuffing. Celebratory and jovial, the parade was nonetheless punctuated by tense moments between residents who support or do not support the copper-nickel-mining plans. At Zaveryl's, a popular spot for locals to drink and watch the parade, the spectators wore pro-mining hats, T-shirts, and stickers. The bar's front window displayed a pro-mining banner. And when the Campaign to Save the Boundary Waters marched by carrying signs about saving the Boundary Waters, the crowd outside Zaveryl's booed and shouted at the marchers, "Go back to the city!" "You don't live here!" A white woman in her forties, who sat in front of me with her two children, quietly remarked that she bet some of the gray-haired marchers actually *were* "from here." Later, providing a sharp contrast, the Conservationists with Common Sense group, which opposes wilderness protections and motor restrictions in the BWCAW, paraded by in a pickup truck, pulling a motorized fishing boat and displaying pro-mining signs and US flags. The driver waved at the patrons outside Zaveryl's, and they responded with cheers and encouragement. A young dad ran up to the truck, lifting his baby to get a kiss from one of the group's leaders as the parade passed. These scenes demonstrated the perception that pro-mining groups are embedded within the local community while environmentalists are outsiders.

Many "old Elyites" and local political leaders say they do not want an economy dependent on serving these outsiders—tourists and retirees. They want to preserve Ely's working-class way of life and see new mining projects as key to this effort. John, a white man in his early fifties, is a community leader who works in small business and education. He described how copper-nickel mines would help maintain the city's "hardscrabble" character:

> Ely, I think, has to be vigilant to keep its identity. But again, I don't want that identity to change to just be somewhere where a bunch of liberals move to—basically, retired liberals move to make this a liberal, eco-paradise. . . . So many of the local people who have places at Burnside Lake can't afford it. We don't want to move to two classes, where you have those folks that move up here and have multimillion-dollar homes and whatever, and then you have a class of former miners. Now we need some quality jobs for the working people, what America used to have, what Donald Trump ran on.

Trump's campaign message connected with this defensive stance, providing a message of hope about the return to an industrial past for white, working-class, rural people feeling displaced by liberal, urban elites—ironically, the messenger was a millionaire real estate developer and reality-TV star from New York City.

Us-versus-them rhetoric is used to paint environmentalists as outsiders who are both elitists and extremists. This a common tactic used by corporations and anti-environmental movements to discount environmental activists by framing them as dangerous and out of touch, creating divides between workers and environmentalists while presenting a populist image for anti-environmentalism.[26] Copper-nickel-mining supporters regularly described environmentalists as radical, elite, and urban, indicative of how the issue is intertwined with broader political and cultural conflicts across rural-urban and class divides. Framing environmentalists as elitists and extremists is contradictory yet complementary. This relies on one stereotypical image of urban wealthy liberals who want to protect their vacation homes and places for outdoor recreation, along with another image of dirty, dreadlocked young protestors using direct action and violence to stop development. Using both of these tropes enables a flexible discourse to present environmentalists as outsiders who are out of touch with the concerns and values of rural, working-class residents.

Environmentalists were often described as being ideologically opposed to technology and economic growth while not understanding the realities of mining and manufacturing, which are necessary for modern society. Tom, the retired miner and community leader in Ely whom I introduced at the beginning of the chapter, said that many of the environmentalists and other urban and college-educated people opposed to mining are "CAVE people: citizens against virtually everything." Thus, resistance to copper-nickel mining is supposedly irrational and driven by ideology.

Framing environmentalists as outside extremists links copper-nickel-mining debates to fears about supposedly "disruptive" and "violent" protests happening across the US to block oil and gas infrastructure, like the protests over the Keystone XL and Dakota Access Pipelines.[27] In Minnesota, there is an ongoing struggle over Enbridge's Line 3 oil pipeline, which would cross waterways across northern Minnesota and Ojibwe territory. Opponents have formed protest encampments, led marches and protests, and used some direct-action and civil-disobedience tactics.[28] Pro-mining groups attempt to link all of these issues and groups together. However, almost all of the organizations involved in copper-nickel mining are mainstream groups with professional staff who are focused on policy and legal issues. More-radical environmental groups have not been that active, and there have not been direct actions or disruptive protests over copper-nickel mining.

Iron Range politicians and pro-mining activists often blamed "environmental extremists" for divisions in the DFL and for being out of touch with the needs of working-class people—coded as white and rural. At a pro-mining rally, a DFL state legislator from the Iron Range said, "That's why I said extremist versus the environmentalist. I think a lot of people up here would consider themselves the environmentalist with just as much sincerity as anyone else who feels that they can claim that for themselves." This argument deflects responsibility for interparty tensions away from staunchly pro-mining Iron Rangers, while presenting their position as reasonable.

The related tactic of framing environmentalists as elitists also situates copper-nickel mining as a tension between rural and urban residents and between working- and upper-class people. This frame draws on a perception that white, rural, and working-class communities are looked down on by urbanites and environmentalists who do not understand their way of life. An opinion article in the *Mesabi Daily News* written by the president of Up North Jobs, a small pro-mining group in Ely, portrayed Sustainable Ely—the name of the visitor center run by Northeastern Minnesotans for Wilderness and the CSBW—as being backed by people with deep pockets in the city: "With a tiny base of supporters in Ely opposed to mining, Sustainable Ely has begun to shift its effort to the Twin Cities where they find friendly supporters and wealthy friends." The article went on to make a populist claim that mining revenue would benefit everyone, while elites want to stop the project in order to keep the BWCAW for themselves: "The tax and royalty revenues produced by mining are enjoyed by citizens statewide—not just the privileged few who act on the proposition that they are the gatekeepers to control access to the Boundary Waters."[29]

Tony, the union organizer I introduced earlier, lamented upper-class environmentalists in the DFL for pushing people to Trump: "I have some of them as friends, and I said, 'All you're gonna do is succeed in getting Trump people elected, and you won't have anything going for you, period.'" He summed up the pro- and anti-mining tensions this way: "Our cause is to have jobs that can pay people to have a living. Your cause [environmentalists] is, okay, 'We all get to drink water,' but what else? And that's a real struggle in Minnesota. Minnesota could flip real easy, big time, and they're not gonna flip to the correct side. It's gonna flip to the dark side. It almost did up here." Tony, in effect, charged that the wealthy are able to worry about clean water because they are not struggling to make ends meet, a point that overlooks the country's history of working-class environmentalism.[30] The same tradition of unionized laborers fighting against mine bosses and big corporations has also inspired fights to preserve safe drinking water, clean air, and wildlife against reckless waste disposal and other corporate shortcuts for well over a century.

Environmentalists prove a simple and a tangible scapegoat, unlike the abstract and complex forces of global capitalism, industrial policy, and neoliberal retrenchment. Attacking outside extremist and elitist environmentalists allows politicians and corporations to claim that they are on the side of workers and rural communities when the neoliberal policies they often enact are doing much of the harm. Blaming environmentalists diverts responsibility for economic woes away from corporations' reducing labor costs and outsourcing production or the lack of government policies to support rural livelihoods.

At the same time, environmentalists are also culpable in these tensions. Some groups and activists reproduce classist rhetoric about saving wilderness from people who *do not value nature*. A prominent conservation leader in Ely and retired lawyer was quoted in the *New York Times* saying, "They want somebody to just give them a job so they can all drink beer with their buddies and go four-wheeling and snowmobiling with their buddies, not have to think about anything except punching a clock."[31] It would be hard to find a better emblem for the Iron Rangers who suspected they were being judged by upper-class environmentalists, and the article spawned local controversy. Incidents like this are emblematic of how environmental groups struggle to connect with rural and working-class people's experiences or address the issues they care most deeply about.

However, the classist sentiments in the *New York Times* quote were not common in the time I spent with environmentalists, even if some of those attitudes may exist. Environmentalists I spoke with expressed concerns over Iron Rangers' economic struggles and demonstrated an awareness of the class and economic issues at hand in the copper-nickel fights. Brad, a young organizer with the CSBW, remarked that the group does not want to put people out of work but to create an alternative, more prosperous future: "The number-one problem that I always want people to understand—or the miscommunication, I should say, that I want people to understand—is that none of us are trying to put any of these people into negative circumstance. None of us. It's not a matter of me taking away their jobs or taking away their livelihoods. It's a matter of rethinking how we all move forward as a society."

I met Arthur, a former professor, and his wife, an artist, at their house in the woods a few miles outside of Ely, where they recently moved after retiring. Arthur's involvement in environmental groups opposing the Twin Metals project was similarly nuanced. Like Brad, he understood why "old Ely" focused on jobs and why those jobs needed to be stable, long-term, high-paying, and, unlike tourism, year-round: "I'd like to see some sort of really burly job, and I don't think it can be one big industry. But I would like to see some good, strong pursuit of jobs that will not have a boom-and-bust component to them. I mean, I'd like to see more jobs here. I think it's totally valid that the people who want good jobs and want something so the people who were born here could stay here." Environmental groups are often aware and understanding when it comes to the concerns expressed by workers in rural communities, yet they struggle to articulate a convincing, streamlined narrative and concrete proposals to address those concerns. Far too few of the organizations opposing copper-nickel mining are also putting time and resources into promoting just transitions that would help the Iron Range move to a more environmentally sustainable economy without leaving workers behind. Their primary public messaging is about environmental pollution and wilderness conservation, overlooking potentially appealing critiques of corporate power as well as calls for environmental and economic justice for longtime Iron Rangers.

Excessive Government Regulation

The federal government is another of the perceived outside threats facing the Iron Range. Mine supporters lament bureaucratic red tape that has delayed development, constraining locals' livelihoods in the name of environmental protection. This ideology is common in the US, where it is used by anti-environmentalists and right-wing populists to frame environmental regulations as harms to working-class people and as interference in locals' rights to secure their livelihoods.[32] And the logic is effective: it promises that expanding resource extraction and eliminating environmental protections is a populist cause, a way to take back the people's power when it comes to decisions about using the land and resources that constitute their backyard—although it would actually give more power to outside corporations to extract profits from the land.

Corporations, pro-mining leaders, and politicians alike have attributed delays in mining expansions on the Iron Range to excessive regulations and politicized government agencies beholden to environmentalists. In an email newsletter about the PolyMet project's delays, then-congressman Nolan wrote, "Minnesota's Iron Range got a real slap in the face and a punch in the gut by Washington bureaucrats last week. . . . The Washington bureaucrats have clearly overreached their authority."[33] By stoking anger and mistrust against the federal government, Nolan and others help create the unified sense of a community that must defend itself against outsiders. Pro-mining groups picking up on this rhetoric have gone further, promoting the idea that locals are the only true experts on this region and that they support commonsense environmental regulations—they do not need outside interference in order to maintain the pristine waters of northern Minnesota.

Ethan works for the US Forest Service in Ely, an agency that has been subject to a great deal of contention and scrutiny (recall that its office was vandalized during the 1970s BWCAW fights). He described longtime residents' animosity toward the federal government: "I've heard it said recently that we are taking away the minerals that are rightfully theirs, and they're really not. [These resources] are on public land. They're all of ours, and we all decide." In contrast to local residents, Ethan uses wilderness populism framing to claim that the place belongs to all people in the US and that the public lands should be kept public.

Trump's messages about cutting red tape and "draining the swamp" connected with Iron Rangers' resentment toward environmental regulations and expert-led policy, causing even some ardent DFL supporters to throw their support behind the unconventional candidate. Anti-regulation and anti-government discourse from pro-mining Democrats can be puzzling, because this rhetoric aligns with Republican issues like states' rights and small government. One pro-mining activist, a middle-aged white resident, directly told me that the permitting process for a new mine in Minnesota takes too long because there are "too many fingers in the pie" and that it was this frustration that led him and others like him to vote Republican in 2016.

Industry uses the same framing about federal overreach to mobilize support for new mining projects and pro-business policies. Max, a middle-aged representative of a mining industry group, connected anger about the federal government and environmentalists' influence to the 2016 election. During our interview, he described a decision by the US Forest Service under the Obama administration to put a moratorium on mining in the BWCAW watershed this way: "To me it's a perfect example of why Hillary Clinton lost rural America in 2016. It's federal government overreach. It's politically motivated. It's not based on science."

Still, the stances of residents and pro-mining groups on the Iron Range are complex and distinct from other regions in the US. Many express environmental concerns but trust that state regulations and oversight by residents and workers will ensure that copper-nickel mining is clean and safe. Few deny that there are risks, but they think the risks can be managed. This rhetoric is similar to the ways that ranchers and farmers sometimes argue that they—not federal regulators—are best suited to protect the environment because of their hands-on experience with the land and their practical knowledge.[34] This contradictory pro-regulation and pro-environmental framing to justify risky extractive industries is different from other anti-environmental movements that use conventional conservative themes. For example, Arlie Hochschild, a Berkeley sociologist, spent several years in the mid-2010s living with people in a Tea Party stronghold of Louisiana. She found that white and working-class people drew on conservative political ideas about small government and individual responsibility to oppose environmental regulations, despite experiencing public health problems from industrial pollution.[35] In Minnesota, people express concerns about the collective good and think commonsense state regulations are to thank for keeping the region's water clean.

Out-of-Touch Democrats

Often, the mining supporters I met, including local Democratic activists and leaders, expressed anger at the Democratic Party leadership and establishment. They believe the party has drifted from its working-class and labor (implicitly white) base to become a party of the educated elite and urban immigrants and people of color. Defending a rural "us" means, for many, that it is time to give Republican leaders a chance. This reflects a trend among rural residents who see cities as fundamentally different from small towns and see "Washington" as part of the outside, and often urban, forces intervening in rural affairs.[36] In an op-ed for a regional newspaper, a man who identified as an Iron Ranger, a third-generation union member, and a lifelong Democrat wrote, "Not only do the Twin Cities Democrats not care about the Iron Range economy, they actually despise and look down upon us. The time for talking with these people is over. It's time to flip the Range to red and let them know we won't tolerate their anti-mining nonsense. The Iron Range is not going to be their playground."[37]

Elsewhere on the Iron Range, a city council member similarly claimed that he was a lifelong union member and Democrat but shared with me that he had voted for Trump. He thought the Republican candidate stood up for the "working man" and that Democrats and environmentalists had gone too far, "opposing everything," while Trump addressed the important "meat and potatoes" issues that affected people like him. Trump's appeals to stand up for rural and working-class people—implicitly white and often male—by eliminating environmental regulations and restoring mining and manufacturing jobs provided a sense of visibility and pride for people who felt ignored by urban elites, the federal government, and environmentalists seen as controlling the Democratic Party.

This anti-Democrat anger is braided together with racism and xenophobia. Urban-versus-rural divides are often racialized. Right-wing populist politicians' calls to the defend the people are typically coded as a defense of white and rural people.[38] Thus, complaints about the Twin Cities dictating northeastern Minnesotans' way of life were always subtly (and sometimes not so subtly) tied to Iron Rangers' broader racialized sentiments. At a public hearing in Duluth about federal mineral leases for the Twin Metals project, the mayor of Babbitt, a small Iron Range town, contrasted her town's economic struggles with the money and development in Duluth and the Twin Cities and extolled the need to listen to rural people's needs, claiming that "mining lives matter." This reference to the Black Lives Matter movement and the reactionary slogans of "Blue Lives Matter" and "All Lives Matter" explicitly situated the discussion about mining within broader racial and rural-urban politics and white resentment. Supposedly, attention to racial injustice and violence was ignoring the plight of miners, who symbolize rural and white communities.

In my interviews and casual conversations, people spoke reverently about Ely as a safe place to live, the kind of town where people could still leave their doors unlocked and let their kids play outside without supervision. A middle-aged white Elyite claimed that his daughter had moved back to northern Minnesota from the state capital, St. Paul, after enduring too many incidents of cops chasing "thugs" in her alley. The racially coded language of "thugs" presented the city as a racialized and dangerous place, in contrast to safe and white rural towns.

Others harbored resentment that the state's DFL leadership had turned its back on white, working-class, and rural residents in favor of poor, racialized urbanites. For instance, a DFL Minnesota state representative I interviewed made a passing critique of a Latina representative from Minneapolis when discussing the state of the party. He complained that the woman, who had just won a seat formerly held by a longtime white DFL politician, was not actually that progressive and "just turned on her Spanish accent when she wanted to"—implying that she only used her racial and ethnic identity strategically, as ways to advance her political career in a moment when the DFL was targeting communities of color. This comment revealed a broader critique about identity politics and fears that the traditional white power bases in the DFL were losing influence.

Resource Independence and Nationalism

Extractive populism links the defense of local ways of life with defense of the nation. Resource nationalism allows mining proponents to claim that development projects will secure a stable domestic supply of natural resources, thereby reducing foreign dependencies and protecting US security.[39] Miners and rural mining regions are used in this rhetoric as symbols of the people and the nation, embodiments of an idealized heartland and heritage in need of protection.[40]

A common rationale I heard for opening copper-nickel mines is the need for a domestic supply of minerals so the US can be resource independent and not depend on untrustworthy foreign countries such as Russia and China. Max, the spokesperson for an industry group, posed a hypothetical question in our interview: "Where do you want your metals to come from?" His question assumes, a priori, that the sourcing of industrial materials matters, and it implies that US mined metals will actually be used in US products and projects. The retired miner and community leader Randy remarked that the proposed copper-nickel mines would "provide for some of our national security too": "That's a big part of it. Like I said, we import 100 percent of our nickel." Relying on foreign, possibly untrustworthy countries like Russia and China, he argued, makes the US vulnerable, while mining in Minnesota protects the US. It is a handy argument, but it overlooks the fact that copper and nickel are traded on global commodities markets—where the US both buys and sells nickel and copper.

So often, the world today is described as uncertain and changing. Nationalist, protectionist sentiments, on the other hand, offer hope and provide a sense of stability. As the Iron Range deals with the cascading effects of deindustrialization, copper-nickel mining can be effectively framed as bolstering the country's economic stability, competitiveness, and security, adding heft to arguments for opening new mining facilities. A 2008 newsletter from the University of Minnesota Natural Resources Research Institute, an applied research center that works on natural resources and economic development, reported,

> Demand for copper, primarily from the growing nations of China and India, has driven the price up to the point where it's targeted by scrap thieves. Robberies in the Duluth area have been reported in which both operating and abandoned buildings have been stripped of their aluminum, copper wiring and copper pipes. "The key for our region, and for the nation, is that these critical minerals are found in our lands and at levels that can make an impact in the amount of imports that we require to satisfy our nation's needs," said NRRI Center Director Don Fosnacht. "The need is especially acute as we compete with China and India for minerals that all industrial societies require."[41]

If economic growth is stymied by reliance on imported resources and if local crime is linked to the dearth of locally supplied copper, it seems that expanding resource extraction is a commonsense, unquestionable "good." Again, the argument rests on presumptions, including a direct relationship between supply and demand on the price of copper and nickel (regardless of how global commodities prices are shaped by futures markets, speculation, and finance), the specter of losing out to foreign competitors, and the idea that small-scale copper theft is about scarce copper, rather than historically high scrap-metal prices and severe economic need.[42]

Appeals to nationalism tidily evoke fear *and* pride. They resonate with long-standing narratives about the Iron Range providing the materials necessary for the US economy and national security. If Plains-states grain farms can garner respect as the nation's "breadbasket," why should the Iron Range not deserve analogous respect? I regularly heard people say that Minnesota's iron mines "built America" and "won the world wars" by providing the steel for the guns, tanks, and planes that went to war. In an op-ed for a regional newspaper, Cynthia Steine, an activist with the grassroots pro-mining group Fight for Mining Minnesota, laid out a typical narrative: "Minnesota's iron-rich ores played an enormous role in the war effort for both World War I and World War II. By World War II, miners and steel producers had unionized; mines and steel factories worked around the clock, and their contribution to victory was vast and unparalleled. America produced more than 188 million metric tons of steel for the war, and northeastern Minnesota was the single largest provider of raw material for the effort. Victory would not have been possible without Minnesota's contribution."[43] Here, the heroic labor of mine workers is celebrated as a sacrifice for the nation, an effort not only to meet domestic need but to advance US power and protect freedom around the world. The natural conclusion is that opposition to mining expansion is simply unpatriotic.

It cannot be overlooked that nationalist discourses about resource independence repackage racialized and xenophobic fears of unfriendly countries. The preceding quotes are typical, in that they use countries like China, Russia, and India to capture the threat of foreign competition, of developing countries' (especially authoritarian countries') growing populations and industrial capacities, and of nonwhite domination. Tim grew up in the town of Hoyt Lakes, a town built by the Erie Mining Company in the 1950s, and followed in his dad's footsteps to work in the Erie mine. To him, the Iron Range needs the Twin Metals and PolyMet projects if the US hopes to compete with China: "Your grandchildren will be working for the Chinese, and *they* will mine it. Let's look at the world as a whole. When I was in high school, they said one-fifth of the world lived in China. Do you think you're going to be able to hold them people back forever? In my lifetime, they've started getting enough to eat, and they're going to progress. . . . The Chinese will not put up with welfare and all this other bullshit. If you don't make the muster in the morning, son, you ain't eating no rice." His words are plainly racist and xenophobic. The China he evokes is ruthless, driven to expansion and unshackled by human-rights concerns and environmental protections. His Orientalism others Chinese people ("them people"), stereotypes Chinese workers, and casually references the famine they faced under Mao. China serves as a scapegoat for economic struggles and job loss to overseas competition, rather than the multinational mining companies that cut jobs and lowered wages, the corporate-friendly tax and trade policies that enabled offshoring, and global economic restructuring that untethered materials' costs from materials' value.

Adding insult to injury, the emphasis that Tim and other mining supporters place on China is overblown. In 2017, China was only the world's eighth-largest producer of nickel and third-largest producer of copper; several countries with smaller production outputs have larger untapped reserves than China does.[44] As of 2016, China was also the world's largest importer of copper and nickel, and the US exported 62 percent of its annual nickel production and 12 percent of its annual copper production to China.[45] In fact, China's growing demand is often cited as a driver for the relatively high copper prices that, in the early 2000s, made US copper-nickel-mining projects so attractive to investors.[46] It even spurred a boom for Minnesota's iron mines in the same period, because China's expanding construction drove up global steel prices.[47] In many ways, the fortunes of Minnesota miners improve because of, not in spite of, Chinese industrialization and growth.

A further contradiction obscured in the nationalist resource-independence discourse is that mines in Minnesota's Arrowhead are not domestic operations—they are being developed by foreign and multinational corporations. Glencore, a massive Swiss mining corporation that ranks sixteenth among the Global Fortune 500 companies, owns a majority stake in PolyMet.[48] Once operations begin, Glencore will sell and trade the metals it produces on the global commodities and futures markets. Twin Metals is a subsidiary of Antofagasta, a Chilean company that is among the world's leading copper producers. If copper and nickel are mined in northeastern Minnesota, the materials will not flow in a straight line from the mines to US manufacturers and into Americans' homes in the form of consumer goods. That just is not how transnational supply networks and markets work.

Right-wing populists like Trump and mining proponents use nationalist rhetoric that links resource nationalism with a populist anti-globalization message. Opposing free-trade deals and threatening tariffs on foreign steel were key ways that Republicans tapped into working-class and union support. This enabled Trump to claim that he would reshape trade policies in order to benefit American workers and bring back mining and manufacturing jobs. Protectionist anti-globalization rhetoric was particularly effective in the Iron Range because it happened to match up with ongoing debates about protecting the iron industry from foreign competition. Political and union leaders blamed layoffs and closures of Minnesota's iron mines in 2015 and 2016 on the Chinese government's practice of "dumping" artificially low-priced Chinese steel into the US market.[49] Minnesota's legislators, spearheaded by Iron Range Democrats, subsequently pressured the Obama administration to put tariffs on Chinese steel in March 2016, then credited the tariffs with reviving iron production and putting thousands of miners back to work.[50] When DFL congressman Nolan narrowly held onto his seat in 2016, many observers attributed the win to his support for the tariffs. One of his campaign press releases claimed, "That's why some 1,000 Iron Range miners are already back to work. Thanks to these cripplingly high new tariffs and taxes, Range iron prices are up, steel imports are down, the glut of foreign steel is disappearing and America's steel industry—the foundation of our economic and military security—is on the rebound."[51] Obama-era policies may have protected iron-mining jobs in Minnesota. Then, in 2016, the Trump campaign courted union and working-class voters by arguing for a continued need to protect the US steel industry from unfair Chinese competition. Democrats and union leaders were in a complicated position in 2016: they needed to maintain opposition to Trump and cultivate the Democratic voting base, support the sorts of steel tariffs and free-trade critiques credited to Democrats but now claimed by Trump, *and* navigate the association of their presidential candidate, Hillary Clinton, with her husband's presidency and the troubling legacy of North American Free Trade Agreement (NAFTA) free-trade policies.

Interestingly, opponents of Twin Metals counter the pro-mining arguments with their own patriotic framing, presenting public lands and wilderness recreation as important to veterans. The CSBW created the Veterans for the Boundary Waters to demonstrate the diversity of its coalition and appeal to veterans and more conservative people. While chatting with CSBW volunteers at their booth during the Blueberry Arts Festival in Ely, which attracts thousands of people to town every summer, I heard one volunteer talking with an older man with a beard, tattered jeans, and a black veteran's T-shirt. The volunteer thanked him for his service before telling him about the many veterans involved with the campaign to stop mining in the BWCAW watershed. The CSBW argued that the tranquility of wilderness was important in helping veterans heal from the traumas of war but also that unpolluted public lands were necessary for the fishing and hunting that many vets enjoy. Protecting the federal wilderness areas—a symbol of the nation—was thus a patriotic act and a way to respect and honor veterans.

Grassroots Digital Activism and Networking

Support for copper-nickel mining is not only from industry-backed groups or corporate public relations. There are grassroots, pro-mining activists in Minnesota, many of whom are connected through online communities to regional and national networks that promote resource extraction and scaling back environmental regulations. Minnesota Miners, Fight for Mining Minnesota, and other local activists have connected with groups in western states like Arizona, Nevada, and Montana, plugging into the broader conservative states'-rights, small-government, and anti-environmental movement. At the extreme end, these groups are associated with militia groups and figureheads like Ammon Bundy, whose family led an armed takeover of the Oregon Malheur National Wildlife Refuge in 2016 (a follow-up to their 2014 armed standoff resisting the Bureau of Land Management's attempt to collect over $1 million in unpaid federal grazing fees).[52] Online communications and social media were key to making these connections as well as amplifying the voices of more reactionary and conservative activists. Beyond promoting copper-nickel mining, which pro-mining union and DFL leaders also sought, these groups often wanted to shift Iron Range politics to the right.

Online activism helped groups in Minnesota expand their presence and gain attention locally and nationally. Though small and only loosely affiliated, these groups used web-based tactics like swarming politicians' Twitter accounts and hashtags with messages, coordinating comments on Facebook, and creating virtual petitions to embolden supporters and give them an outsized voice. Rob, a fifty-something man who grew up in Ely and recently returned to the area, explained that, although he never worked in the mining industry, he got involved in a grassroots mining group. After some internal disagreements, he left to form his own group. The group specialized in using social media to share information and pressure elected officials. As Rob put it in our conversation, Twitter is the group's major tool, and it tweeted regularly at people like the secretaries of the interior and agriculture, politicians from the Western Caucus (a group of Republican congresspeople from western states and rural areas), and specific politicians from Minnesota, Arizona, and Arkansas who are involved with mining issues. Rob went on to explain, "We do it on a daily basis. All these people follow us. They're actually seeing all the tweets we're putting out. I'd like to believe to a certain extent that we've had some influence on what's been going on." The apparently direct access to power players helped Rob feel that he too could make things happen in US politics.

Steve, who is around Rob's age and was raised near Ely, works in tourism and outdoor recreation, but he is an adamant supporter of copper-nickel mining. He even helped start another pro-mining group. In our interview, he described hatching his plan to organize through social media: "I'm gonna start a Facebook group. I'm gonna try to get three hundred people together, and we're gonna Twitter-bomb Trump. We're gonna speak the language of Trump. I said, he's on Twitter every five minutes. It's all I ever hear about. I don't know much about Twitter, but I'm gonna go.'" Steve was not very politically active before this, but the copper-nickel-mining issue sparked his passion, and his group's vocal online presence got the attention of politicians and reporters, despite his lack of organizing experience or ties to existing organizations. Quickly, he became a prominent figure, regularly quoted in news articles and invited to meetings with state and federal politicians. A normal person like him, he emphasized, could have a voice through Twitter, even without powerful connections.

Many times, social media activism is associated with left-wing causes and youth movements, but anti-environmental activists and older and rural people are building alliances and making connections across the country's regions and communities using digital activism. Their online networks have facilitated the spread of right-wing ideas and political tactics. That is how Iron Range grassroots pro-mining groups have come to share news articles from right-wing sources such as the *Free Range Report*, a libertarian website focused on private-property rights and fights over land and natural resources in the West. In part, this is how the right-wing rhetoric of federal overreach, excessive regulation, and anti-elitism has been attached to support for copper-nickel mining. And that is how money and tactics have flowed from groups struggling to open public lands in the west for resource extraction and national conservative groups into the Iron Range's mining fights. Rob's recollection of plugging his local group into a nationwide conservative network is instructive:

> We started tweeting the people in the Western Caucus at the very beginning when we started in April, because I knew what was going on out there, that they've been fighting this fight for a lot longer than us. They've been fighting the US Forest Service and the BLM [the federal Bureau of Land Management] for decades out there: grazing rights, water rights, things like that. They're saying, "Well, you know what? You guys are basically fighting the same fight that we've been fighting for decades. So you know what? We're going to throw our hat in the ring, and we're going to help you."

The rise of these right-wing pro-mining groups and online networks is interconnected with the ongoing political realignment on the Iron Range. For example, Rob described being a conservative independent who was excited by the Republicans and Trump in 2016. Another local mining activist, Carl, spoke about his active support for Trump, including online promotion of his candidacy.

Other local pro-mining activists told me that the mining industry and unions were not doing enough to promote the copper-nickel proposals. Rob, the self-described conservative independent who had never worked in mining, was not a union member and found it confusing that the unions were not throwing all of their weight behind the proposed copper-nickel mines: "I haven't quite understood why [the labor unions have] been so standoffish. Though I've talked to some union members, and they said, 'Well, it really doesn't affect us.' It's like, 'Well, it could in the long term, though.' If they [environmentalists] win this, who do you think that they're going to go after next?" Rob argued that pro-mining, pro-Trump activists like himself were the true defenders of the Iron Range way of life.

Social media has inarguably changed political organizing and activism, enabling people to communicate without formal organizations and to form new networks for sharing information and tactics.[53] Grassroots pro-mining activists expressed a sense that they are underdogs, fighting without the resources and connections of environmental organizations or unions but successfully and resourcefully using social media to amplify their voices. Several pro-mining activists I spoke with told me that their opponents, the environmentalists, have national political connections and the money to lobby in Washington, DC, while they have to use online strategies. It struck me that their groups are nonetheless working on behalf of a wealthy, powerful industry whose extensive political connections and armies of lobbyists far outpace that of environmental groups. A single example evidences their unparalleled access and influence: public records show that, in 2017, representatives of Twin Metals and its parent company, Antofagasta, met twice with the Department of the Interior's principal deputy solicitor, shortly before he issued a decision renewing Twin Metals' federal mineral leases.[54]

Social media is also contributing to combative rhetoric and escalated conflicts between people on different sides of the mining issue. Patricia, a young organizer with an environmental group, noted that her opponents are getting more organized through online actions: "The pro-copper-mining faction wasn't very organized, and actually, in just the past few months, they've become much more organized. They formed a Facebook group. . . . They organized. The language they use is very aggressive. . . . They troll on Twitter." She elaborated, indicating that online interactions seem to lower inhibitions and encourage confrontation, compared to in-person arguments: "Prior to this, the reaction was always, 'I know this person. They know me.' Maybe it's cordial, face to face, but then when push comes to shove, say, at like a St. Louis County

Commissioner's meeting, I'm gonna say one thing looking at you, and you're gonna say another thing looking at me. I've never been personally attacked. But now with this particular group, it just feels so much more loaded."

A young Elyite who is opposed to copper-nickel mining and who works for a small outdoor-clothing company told me much the same: "To see some of the cyberbullying that's happening in these smaller communities and the power of social media on small-town businesses—we've had some pretty nasty things that people said in reviews on our Yelp account who've never purchased gear from us, who just do it because they say we hate mining." A mix of social media, caustic political divisions, and resurgent authoritarian right-wing politics has contributed to a tense, conflictual climate and a rupture to the civility of small-town communities.

Political Contradictions and Challenges

The anti-environmental, pro-mining rhetoric adopted by many DFL politicians in northeastern Minnesota creates contradictions because it aligns with Republican messaging and platforms. Just like their Republican counterparts, DFL politicians—especially when attacked for not representing "working people"—use combative us-versus-them rhetoric and appeals to romantic nostalgia when they blame urbanites and environmentalists for the problems facing Iron Rangers, rather than blaming corporations and neoliberal policies. Writing in the *Star Tribune*, a journalist reported from the Iron Range, "'We are going to go through some hard times,' predicted Rep. Tom Anzelc, DFL-Balsam Township. 'This may be the signature event in the decades long battle between jobs and the preservation of the environment. This battle determines what kind of a Minnesota Minnesotans want.'"[55]

Tom Rukavina, the influential DFL former state representative and St. Louis County commissioner mentioned earlier, was also quoted by the *Star Tribune*: "'I just wish one day that our good DFL senators, both of them, you know, would tell the environmentalists to quit crying wolf, you can't be against everything,' he said. 'You can't want a broadband if there is no copper. . . . So, cut the crap and grow up.'"[56] Tidily, he accused his colleagues of magical thinking—believing that they could guarantee broadband internet access for the Iron Range even without mining the resources needed to build the infrastructure—and scolded that the logical politician would instead support the mining industry.

Problematically, with messaging that echoes Republicans' pro-business, deregulatory agenda and Trump's right-wing populist discourse, DFL politicians struggle to provide a clear rationale for why people should support the party's candidates, especially at the national level. The 2016 and 2020 election results attest that Iron Range voters split their ballots, voting for DFL candidates for local office but Republican candidates for national roles. Trump won in the region in 2016, as did the incumbent US representative, Nolan, and a host of other DFL politicians running in Minnesota's state and local races.

Iron Rangers who are committed to progressive issues and the DFL are aware of these tensions, worrying openly about what copper-nickel mining might mean for regional politics in the long run and how to keep the region voting blue. I met mining supporters who remained staunch Democrats, despite critiquing the environmental wing of the party. In a response to the op-ed quoted earlier, a union member from the Iron Range wrote that, rather than supporting Republicans, fellow locals must avoid the trap of voting solely on the copper-nickel-mining issue. Republicans, he claimed, may support mining proposals, but they also support policies to weaken unions and workplace protections and give tax cuts to the wealthy.[57]

Plenty of the union activists I met were highly critical of Trump and Republicans, and they wanted to maintain the region's progressive politics while supporting copper-nickel mining. Tony and his parents welcomed me to their 1950s rambler home in Babbitt, a small town built by a mining company. The parents, a retired iron miner and his politically active wife (a member of the local chapter of Indivisible, a national grassroots organization that formed to resist the Trump administration), were in their late seventies, and their son Tony was a union organizer in his fifties. As we chatted in the living room, I learned that the whole family was adamantly opposed to Trump and dismayed at what they saw as a hard rightward political swing in their area. Their concurrent support for the copper-nickel mines was tempered by concerns about the projects' environmental impacts, with Tony and his father lamenting that iron-mining companies had failed on the upkeep of their facilities—corporations, they charged, will always do the bare minimum, putting laborers and nearby residents at risk. They felt strongly that the copper-nickel mines must move forward with strong regulatory enforcement and oversight.

Construction and mining unions are also trying to walk a narrow line, both critiquing Democrats who do not support copper-nickel mining and attempting to convince their members to vote Democrat. Some of these pro-mining unions use us-versus-them framing and emotional and nostalgic rhetoric as they take aim at opponents, including Democrats who oppose copper-nickel mining or suggest tighter regulatory scrutiny. Emil Ramirez, director of United Steelworkers District 11, wrote in an op-ed for the *Duluth News Tribune*, "At a time when too many families live with employment insecurity, we cannot allow this rare opportunity to create family-supporting, community-sustaining jobs slip away. With a viable business plan, a skilled workforce, and a market that has found its footing, we have confidence in NorthMet and sincerely believe in the project's ability to deliver on its promise of a more prosperous future in an environmentally responsible manner."[58] Union leadership—especially at the national level—backed Clinton in the 2016 presidential election, while still using Trump's populist rhetoric. Chris Johnson, president of USW Local 2705, acknowledged the contradiction, telling *Politico* that it was Trump who co-opted union messaging to court the union's workers. Johnson continued, saying that Trump was "not pro-labor" and explaining, "He basically stole the union's message and is using that, but to his core, he doesn't believe any of the stuff we do, but he knows he's getting votes for it."[59]

Union positions on copper-nickel mining are also complex. The most vocal supporters of copper-nickel mining are construction unions, whose largely white and male members could get jobs building the mines. Construction unions tend to be among the most conservative in the US labor movement.[60] PolyMet has already agreed to a project labor agreement (PLA) guaranteeing prevailing wages and the hiring of union contractors. The USW represents iron-mine workers in northern Minnesota and could *potentially* organize workers operating the copper-nickel mines, but without a similar guarantee that permanent mine-operation jobs will be union jobs, it has voiced more muted support than construction unions have. Glencore, the multinational corporation financing PolyMet, has a track record of poor labor practices and contentious relationships with unions, while the USW is a progressive, national union that advocates for economic justice, worker health and safety, labor environmentalism, and new organizing strategies.[61] They are not natural bedfellows.

The labor movement is also contending with divides between the construction and mining unions on the Iron Range and in rural Minnesota and service, health care, and education unions, whose membership dominates labor politics in the Twin Cities and other metropolitan areas. These nonindustrial unions, which represent more women, people of color, and immigrants, strongly rejected the nativist, racist, and sexist policies of Trump and right-wing populism. Yet they have been generally silent on the issue of copper-nickel mining. Even tepid warnings from unionized nurses and physicians regarding the potential public health impacts of copper-nickel mining have generated conflict within the labor movement.[62] At the national level, more-conservative unions whose members work in energy-intensive and extractive industries have struggled with more progressive and social-movement-oriented service-sector unions that are active on climate and racial justice.[63] No one in Minnesota is particularly eager to take a firm stance on an issue that could fracture union solidarity any further.

Conclusion

Proponents of copper-nickel mining use the discourse of *extractive populism* to acknowledge people's sense of powerlessness, anger, and loss; to provide a target for their disenchantment (environmentalists and environmental regulations); and to present a hopeful vision, a return to the nostalgic heyday of mining, in which communities were supported by white masculine labor. When these activists speak of "bringing back mining," it resonates. It feels like a culturally meaningful solution to deindustrialization and the global economic changes that have disrupted the rural moral economy of the Iron Range. Further, it promises that opening up public land for private resource extraction defends the American people against outsiders, whether it is industrializing countries in the Global South, elite environmentalists, or urban communities of color.

Extractivism, anti-environmentalism, and resource nationalism are common discourses in contemporary right-wing populism not only because the mining industry holds political-economic power but because it also holds cultural and symbolic power. It evokes the "heartland" and "the common man" that right-wing populists claim to represent.[64] Yet at the same time that right-wing populists sell policies as benefits to rural and poor communities, their pro-business and deregulatory policies accelerate the processes that create economic hardships in rural and industrial regions.[65] Extractive populism motivates voters on an emotional level, leaving harmful corporate strategies, like eliminating and deskilling labor and avoiding environmental and labor protections, unexamined.

The promise of new mining jobs is also appealing because few other tangible alternatives are on offer. Environmentalists and urban progressives have failed to put forward compelling and culturally meaningful visions of just economic transitions for rural extractive regions. There are few government programs to create decent jobs in more socially and ecologically sustainable industries, and there is a long history of workers and communities being left behind after industrial closures.

I cannot claim to have covered all the factors shaping the rightward shift and the results of the 2016 US election in the region. Still, I argue that copper-nickel mining is a crucial piece of the puzzle when it comes to the Iron Range's swing to the right. Entwined with class and rural-urban tensions, Trump's extractive populist message featured anti-elitism, energy dominance, and a promised return to (white) Americans flourishing. It tapped into the framing that copper-nickel supporters were already using in Minnesota and gave it more heft. It also used environmental regulations and wealthy environmentalists as symbols of the dangers posed by government bureaucracy, experts lacking common sense, and out-of-touch urban liberal elites.

At the same time, any willingness to actively, or at least tacitly, support Trump required voters to accept or dismiss his racist, xenophobic, homophobic, and sexist attitudes and policy proposals. Whiteness gave Iron Range residents cover, the privilege to present their votes for Trump as not racist but economic and cultural and to ignore or even support his anti-immigrant, anti-Black, and misogynistic words and deeds. It also allowed wealthy, urban, white voters pushing right-wing agendas to fund Trump's campaign while claiming that he represented and was elected by the rural working class—a liminal stance that would allow for both claiming credit and deflecting blame, depending on the shifting political winds.[66]

Still, the rightward swing in Minnesota was not simply an embrace of Trump's brand of right-wing populism or ideological manipulation of working-class people. The shift was helped along by changes in the national Democratic Party and the state DFL, both moving toward the interests of their urban, upper-class, and financial constituencies—"the New Democratic Party," personified by Hillary Clinton.[67] Copper-nickel-mining advocates, including Democrats from the Iron Range, argued that a vote for Trump in 2016 was a justifiable rejection of Clintonian politics, rather than a complete embrace of Trump's agenda. One pro-mining activist in Ely even claimed that his opposition to elitist Democrats pushed him to vote for Trump: "It had nothing to do with Trump. Right? It had to do with you guys [Democrats] hardening my position not to be with you." Insofar as the 2016 election was partially a broader reaction against the status quo and elites and given that the progressive populist Bernie Sanders actually defeated the centrist Hillary Clinton in the state's 2016 Democratic primary, it was never inevitable that Trump would gain the support of northeastern Minnesota. In the 2016 Republican primary in Minnesota, after all, Trump had taken third, after Marco Rubio and Ted Cruz. It was only later in Trump's campaign that he emphasized populist and economic issues that resonated in northeastern Minnesota, particularly opposition to free trade and support for imposing tariffs on Chinese steel imports. Having met a number of people who supported Sanders in the primary and then voted for Trump in the 2016 general election, as well as Sanders supporters who declined to vote, I venture that populist sentiments could yet be mobilized to rebuild the Iron Range's leftist legacy.

Conclusion

The accelerating need for metals and minerals to fuel global capitalism and the depletion of existing reserves has raised the stakes for regions grappling with decisions about extractive development. Corporations see the opportunity to extract profits from unearthing materials from the ground and transforming them into commodities. Yet the often-risky methods used to dig up the earth mean that human and nonhuman life is jeopardized and workers and surrounding communities face exploitation and pollution. Thus, conflicts around new sites for resource extraction are roiling communities around the globe, particularly when companies want to turn public land and park and conservation areas into industrial landscapes. At the same time, in the US, where the broader national economy has shifted away from production and manufacturing and toward service and finance, the social and economic fabric of industrial towns has been rewoven in the past fifty years.[1] Some of these towns, like those in northern Minnesota's Iron Range, have gotten by with dwindling mining operations supplemented by tourism revenues; but now, new extractive projects promise a return to the heyday of mining prosperity, with industrial jobs supporting male breadwinners, while also threatening the natural environment and outdoor recreation within it. Economic decline and ruptures to the old moral economy, along with the weakening of unions, have also contributed to the rise of right-wing populism, which points the blame at immigrants, people of color, urbanites, and environmentalists.

By examining one such conflict in rural northern Minnesota, we can see how these controversial decisions go beyond scientific assessments and economic calculations. They are struggles over place, identity, justice, and rights, animated by forces of capitalism, settler colonialism, whiteness, and masculinity that affect politics and social movements beyond any single space. In Minnesota, mining's opponents and proponents alike draw on emotional connections to history and place, as well as hopeful visions of the future, in assessing the risks posed by new copper-nickel-mining projects. Thus, they seek to frame their positions in ways that are legitimate and authoritative. Mining, wilderness areas, lakes, and public lands all carry powerful cultural meanings that evoke emotional reactions; groups across political, class, and rural-urban spectrums mobilize these symbols in their divergent discourses of extractive and wilderness populism.

Proponents of mining often engage collective memories and future imaginaries that celebrate masculine labor, valorize the moral worth of white rural communities, and speak to racialized anxieties about social and demographic change and foreign threats. The region's enduring conflicts, positioned for the public as fights over jobs and the environment, are not simply the result of corporations manipulating workers or ideological obfuscation. They reflect the real and consequential ways people create meaning and construct identity within (and sometimes against) the context of dominant culture, language, and ideology. While my analysis has focused on culture and identities, the political-economic conditions of disinvestment, automation, and precarity create conditions in which polluting industries can exploit "job blackmail."[2] Towns need revenue, jobs, and residents. Promises to renew a prosperous past are enticing offers of security in a time of global insecurity and neoliberalism that offers little social support and few alternatives for rural mining regions.

Environmentalists, for their part, have successfully raised public concern and intervened in regulatory processes to turn a relatively low-key issue—a pair of proposals for a new type of mining in one of the largest mining regions in the US—into a major controversy. They have delayed development as they mobilized to defend a place they see as threatened by an industry that is known to pollute waterways and damage ecosystems, in part by drawing on scientific evidence but more crucially by appealing to local history and imaginaries tied to place. When a mine threatens a cherished wilderness recreation area, its opponents try to connect with memories of outdoor recreation and hopes for preserving tranquil wilderness for future generations to enjoy. This wilderness nostalgia appeals, in particular, to middle-class and white ways of relating to nonhuman nature. When a different mine threatens larger, downstream communities, nearer existing industry and less likely to affect recreation, the groups use public health framing and populist critiques of foreign corporations. For all groups, protecting the sky-blue waters of Minnesota from pollution is a compelling message with cultural resonance.

As conflicts over copper-nickel mining escalated in Minnesota, people were forced to choose sides. The complexity of individuals' identities and views were obviated by a clear binary: pro- or anti-mining. Stereotypes of uneducated and unsophisticated rural workers or elite environmentalists reify static social categories and prevent the formation of coalitions that might fight, together, for environmental and economic justice. The categories of worker and environmentalist, old-timer and newcomer, are, at the individual level, rather complex and fluid, yet they have social power. Their boundaries snap shut when political leaders and activists draw on these identities during conflicts, and these identities resonate with broader rural-urban and class divisions in US politics.

Through an analysis of the cultural politics of mining, I push environmental sociology and social movement studies to address the role of memory, emotion, and place in contested politics. In doing so, I build on the environmental sociologist Kari Norgaard's research on the role of emotions in people's understandings and collective denial of environmental problems to show the ways that affective meanings of place and collective memory shape both active acceptance and resistance to environmentally risky industries.[3] How the history of a place is remembered and how its future is imagined are important dynamics in political struggles, especially when it comes to the balance of conservation and industrial development.

Notions of "justice" are just as variegated as identities. My case study demonstrates the need for environmental justice scholarship to examine the tensions and contradictions in the perception of justice across intersecting lines of class, race, gender, indigeneity, and rurality. For instance, job blackmail plays out differently in rural versus urban communities and in white communities versus communities of color: there are lots of reasons that residents may invite risky, profit-seeking industries into their backyards. On the Iron Range, white and working-class residents frame mining opposition as a form of injustice, with elites arriving to threaten their livelihoods and community. Their support for the Twin

Metals and PolyMet proposals is often presented as a defense of their community and their rights (and backyards) against outsiders' attempts to choose what happens (in a place that is only their playground). Conservationists and outdoor-recreation enthusiasts, who are largely white, middle class, and suburban or urban, instead interpret development as an injustice that threatens their aesthetic and emotional connections to the land. Other mining-opposed environmental groups see their work as a justice endeavor in standing up for public health and clean water against the interests of multinational corporations. And Native American tribes and Indigenous activists, for their part, argue against new mining as a potential violation of treaty rights and a further rupture to their long-standing ethical and just relationships with nonhuman nature.

Sociology has traditionally focused on political, economic, and cultural systems to explain social phenomena, but these must be understood in relationship to biophysical systems and the entanglements of human and nonhuman life. As the sociologists William Freudenberg, Scott Frickel, and Robert Gramling contend in an influential article, nature and society are mutually constituted.[4] Thus, my case is instructive in offering a comparison between two types of mining and two different mine locations. Biophysical factors shape sociopolitical reactions to specific types and sites of resource extraction. The geochemistry of copper and nickel ores create additional pollution risks compared to iron ores. And the specific location of different proposed copper-nickel mines leads to different regulatory responses and sociocultural understandings of the projects—one impacting a wilderness area and another impacting larger downstream and Indigenous communities. These differences have generated divergent movement strategies and priorities that reflect tensions within environmental and conservation movements, in which white, urban, and middle-class activists focus on preserving nature and maintaining an idealized wilderness, pushing out or even criminalizing the ways that rural, white, and working-class and Indigenous people use the same land.[5] Deeper attention to culture and biophysical processes will move environmental sociology in new directions and engage transdisciplinary conversations about the complexities of society-nature relations and global environmental problems.

Political Rifts and Corporate Legitimacy

The political and practical implications of my research are not unequivocal, though I can offer fruitful suggestions for understanding and working to overcome class and rural-urban divisions, as well as conflicts between labor and the environment. Examining the rightward swing in northern Minnesota helps untangle contemporary political divisions and reconfigure what we know about building political coalitions that might advance socioenvironmental justice. And looking beyond the Iron Range gives perspective to the broader implications of studying power, culture, and ideology in the contested politics of resource extraction and environmental protection.

Conflicts over the environment are often overlooked among the multiple factors behind the gradual breakdown in the postwar liberal Democratic political alliance of urban progressives, industrial workers, and communities of color.[6] Environmentalism has come to symbolize the elitism of urban liberals and out-of-touch bureaucrats—a disregard for the livelihoods of troubled industrial and extractive regions. Using this narrative, Republicans claim that the Democratic Party has strayed from its working-class and rural base. In combination with various racist and nativist appeals, this rhetoric has been effective at pulling in white, rural, and working-class voters in places like Wisconsin, Ohio, and, increasingly, Minnesota.[7] Right-wing extractive populism speaks to people's identities and emotions, and it provides a clear solution and promise of stability amid economic, social, and political change. The "smokestack nostalgia" that I have traced throughout this book presents mining as inextricable from the vitality of these communities—and its haze constrains alternative imaginaries.[8] Extractive populism links mining to notions of modernity and the good life and is a symbol of the nation and its people; thus, expanding extraction is framed as a patriotic defense of the people and rural values against elitist environmentalism and foreign threats.

In a neoliberal era of rising precarity and inequality, shrinking corporate taxes and public services, and accelerating socioenvironmental crises, the old methods of sustaining consent and legitimacy for resource-intensive and polluting capitalism may be weakening. People are living with the daily realities of the climate crisis: supersized storms and extreme weather, historic droughts, and dirty air. Job blackmail should not work as well when there are fewer and worse jobs and little public revenue to promise, especially when weighed against the often grave ecological and health risks. And so cultural, ideological, and emotional appeals gain significance for pro-mining factions hoping to secure and sustain legitimacy. Mining corporations cannot deny automation (which undermines employment potential) or that they are pursuing low-grade resources using riskier technologies in often remote areas. Government's and corporations' emotional appeals to place and class identities and nostalgia are perhaps the best tactic they have left.[9]

When a community's collective identity is linked to a single, economically dominant industry, PIMBY politics are no surprise, despite environmental risks. Therefore, regions with a history of resource extraction and a strong community economic identity may provide attractive sites for extractive investment—these are excellent predictors for where industry can secure what it calls the "social license to operate."[10] Mining and fossil fuel companies are well aware of the resistance posed by workers and communities in the Global South, especially where the livelihoods of agricultural, subsistence, and Indigenous communities are put at risk.[11] That heightens the attractiveness of sites in the Global North, where mining legacies smooth over local resistance, even if this means contending with relatively higher labor costs and stronger environmental protections.[12] In the US, the attractiveness of historical mining regions for new development also coincides with nationalist political support for extraction as a way to secure resource and energy independence. Republicans and Democrats alike use this justification: as many observers rightly note, President Barack Obama championed the domestic oil and gas fracking boom.[13]

However, there are always competing understandings of place. Extractive industries must work to suppress resistance and sustain their dominant vision for the landscape. Resistance to extractive development arises when protected and cherished places are threatened and industrialization expands to new areas, encroaching on recreation areas and Indigenous territory. Environmental groups are able to drum up opposition, for instance, to the Twin Metals mine by making appeals to wilderness nostalgia, the cultural discourses of a Minnesotan collective identity bound to fishing, outdoor recreation, and the pristine waters of this Land of 10,000 Lakes.

Both sides set themselves up as the "real protectors" of the place. Mining companies and pro-mining unions and Iron Range residents and community leaders frame mining as compatible with a clean environment and safe water—that if the lakes are pristine now, after over a century of iron mining, they will remain so, particularly because modern mining is all about corporate sustainability. Like other industries, it has appropriated environmental rhetoric through greenwashing, including claims to conduct rigorous scientific analysis, adhere to intensive regulatory scrutiny, and implement cutting-edge technologies that ensure safety.[14] The mining industry's so-called corporate social responsibility efforts over the past several decades have helped craft the image of a modern, high-tech, and environmentally responsible industry. This appeals to an ecomodern masculinity that expresses concern for protecting the environment through technological ingenuity and market mechanisms.[15] Greenwashing allows mine supporters to argue that copper, nickel, and other metals are actually necessary for the green economy and forward-thinking energy transitions.[16] As the scale of ecological crises grows and people confront the consequences of pollution, resource depletion, and human and nonhuman exploitation, the rhetoric of environmentalism and science gives cover to the very forces that produce those crises.

Corporate public-relations strategies would not, however, be effective in gaining support for copper-nickel mining on the Iron Range if they did not resonate with locals' own meaning-making processes and relationships to the place. Interestingly, I do not find that Iron Rangers employ the conservative and libertarian rhetoric that other researchers have found, particularly in southern states, among white and working-class people promoting industry and opposing environmentalism.[17] Local stances are complex and ambiguous, with even mine supporters in Minnesota demanding that companies prove the safety of their projects and that regulatory bodies strictly enforce labor and environmental measures. The frictions encountered by global capital in every corner are affected by the place-based historical and political-economic contexts that shape how individuals and communities react to industrial development.[18]

Alternative Possibilities and Alliances

Policies to promote capitalist extractive development and roll back environmental protections will ultimately exacerbate the same processes that have created the economic dislocation that conservative politicians and corporations leverage in rural and industrial regions like the Iron Range. Extractive capitalism relies on finite resources—both those it aims to extract and the fossil fuels that power the extraction (and in turn the climate crisis). Automation and new technologies mean that the same industries require less labor, and the need for high-skilled workers often means importing laborers rather than hiring them locally. Fundamentally, that is, extractivism rests on capitalist, colonialist, and racist logics that devalue human labor as well as nonhuman nature. Its systems create pollution, waste, and exploitation. It cannot ensure the economic, physical, and social well-being of rural and working-class communities or avert ecological crises arising from the socioenvironmental contradictions of capitalism.

Most mainstream environmental organizations opposing copper-nickel mining have struggled to craft a vision for alternative economies that resonates with blue-collar workers and rural residents. Instead of emphasizing economic issues, just transitions for mining workers and communities, or broader issues of socioenvironmental justice, they have focused on technocratic politics, such as submitting scientific comments on environmental impact assessments and litigation and appeals to wilderness nostalgia. Claiming that science and experts "prove" that mining is dirty is not effective messaging for bridging class, rural-urban, and other social divides. It creates barriers to collaboration with workers, unions, and other social justice movements. For example, the anti–Twin Metals events I attended in Minneapolis at a Patagonia store and a microbrewery were populated by white and middle-class outdoor-recreation enthusiasts. Nowhere did I see the cities' vibrant social movements, whose members were so visible and diverse at the marches, rallies, and direct actions around opposition to the Dakota Access Pipeline, in resistance to Trump's anti-immigrant policies, and in support of the Black Lives Matter movement following the police killings of Jamar Clark in 2015 and Philando Castile in 2016 in the Twin Cities. All this political struggle was happening at the same time, but the groups working on copper-nickel mining largely appeared to lack the cross-coalitional imagination of the other struggles.

In particular, the groups focused on Twin Metals have neglected appeals to environmental justice and alternative development and just transitions. In doing so, they have reinscribed the idea that environmentalism is a middle-class, elite, white concern. These organizations often highlight the economic benefits of tourism, arguing that copper-nickel mining is economically detrimental on the grounds that it pollutes nature and deters visitors. Though tourism *may* actually generate more jobs and revenue than mining (at least in the part of the Iron Range nearest the BWCAW), these appeals hold little water with longtime residents, mining and construction workers, unions, or the Iron Range cities and towns that *are not* tourist destinations, where locals yearn for higher-paying, culturally meaningful jobs doing industrial, manufacturing, and manual labor or careers in growth sectors like education and health care.[19]

Identities and emotional ties to place may make conservation/extraction conflicts intractable, but these divisions are not inevitable. Alternatives are possible. Unions and workers, even in mining, are not inherently opposed to environmental protections.[20] For example, the historian Chad Montrie documents how some members and leaders of the United Mineworkers of America opposed ecologically damaging strip mining and sought to align with environmentalists against the coal industry.[21] Populism can be progressive, building labor-environment alliances that challenge elite politicians and corporations while promoting an equitable, sustainable, and democratic economy—US history is full of examples, including, in Minnesota, resistance to NAFTA and free trade.[22] Remember that the Democrats in Minnesota belong to the Democratic-Farmer-Labor Party, created by the 1944 merger of the Democratic and Farmer-Labor Parties, which reflects the state's history of urban-rural alliances and leftist populism.[23] In the 1940s and '50s, the United Steelworkers and other industrial unions opposed Reserve Mining Company's practice of dumping iron tailings into Lake Superior on the grounds that it damaged the environment and public health while also allowing Reserve Mining to cut jobs.[24] The 2006 founding of the Blue Green Alliance brought together the USW and the Sierra Club in an effort spurred by Minnesota's USW District 11 executive director

David Foster to advance labor-environment collaboration around issues like green job creation and climate change. It has been the growing tensions over copper-nickel mining and oil and gas pipelines that have weakened these labor-environment alliances, but these coalitions can be reinvigorated and reimagined.[25]

To begin making, or repairing, cross-movement and cross-regional alliances will require tangible and robust plans to create more sustainable industries at the scale necessary to address unemployment, poverty, and declining and aging populations. The solution cannot be tourism or teleworking alone, because many rural residents who want good jobs with meaningful work will be left out. Being a canoe guide or salesperson at an outdoor store, a largely seasonal, low-skill, low-pay job, does not compare for Iron Rangers with the cultural meaning, pay, and benefits of the union mining jobs they remember (or understand through regional collective memories). As an Ely city councilwoman told me, "You cannot live on a tourist job up here."

So what would justice mean for those who stand to lose jobs as the economy is decarbonized and transformed to be less resource intensive? Just transition is a concept that was initially developed by labor unions in the 1970s, which called for assistance to displaced workers and communities facing industry closures. They argued that workers should not bear the brunt of the burden from closing polluting and outdated facilities. The concept has gained popularity and traction since the 2010s and become part of the global climate change discourse that is used by social movements, front-line communities, politicians, international organizations, and even industry.[26] In the Iron Range, there are no workers who stand to lose existing jobs should copper-nickel mining be blocked (though, to mining hopefuls, it certainly feels that way). Nonetheless, the region needs a transition away from its legacy extractive economy and toward different but sustainable livelihoods. Just transition programs might involve public investments in developing alternative industries, such as manufacturing green-energy materials and outdoor-recreation equipment, health care, and education, as well as funding the necessary social and physical infrastructure, such as job-training programs in community colleges and broadband internet. Jobs could be created cleaning up the environment and remediating industrial and mining facilities rather than opening more land to extraction and subsequent degradation. Just transition programs and advocates must take heed that a job is more than a paycheck—all people want culturally meaningful and fulfilling work. Thus, new jobs need to speak to people's labor and place-based identities. Nor can these solutions be crafted by policy makers and experts behind closed doors, or they will be regarded with the same suspicion attending "outsider" interventions; participatory decision-making will help ensure that people have a voice in crafting the future of their communities. Through public and collective deliberation, people can begin to imagine a future that moves beyond extraction and exploitation of both nonhuman nature and human labor.

Language also matters. How environmentalists talk about issues, from alternative economic development to the risks of mining, is important for bridging social divides. Efforts to create working-class support for environmentalism, for instance, will fail without compelling visions of the future that do not disparage the legacy of mining but instead draw on values of solidarity, hard work, and economic justice. On the Iron Range, this may mean connecting with counternarratives that are critical of industry, including collective memories of mine workers' resistance and organizing, past occupational hazards and exploitative labor conditions, and distrust toward large, outside corporations. These narratives disrupt the romance of smokestack nostalgia while sidestepping potentially divisive wilderness nostalgia frames, which bring defensive responses by invoking outsiders and elites. This would help direct animosity toward the true elites and powerbrokers: mining CEOs and global investors.

A few environmentalists I interviewed said that they were attempting to build bridges with unions, including the USW, which is leading a global campaign in Canada and Colombia against PolyMet's main investor, Glencore, over human rights, labor, and environmental abuses, by questioning the company's labor practices.[27] But my interviews revealed that pro-mining Iron Rangers dismiss such critiques on the basis of their trust that the copper-nickel operations really will bring good jobs back and their distrust of environmental groups. PolyMet *has* agreed to hire union workers to build its facility, an assurance that has gone lengths in getting the support of construction unions and building locals' trust, but few seem to question who will be hired to run the mine once it is built—there is no guarantee that those workers will be unionized or even local.[28]

Another area for possible collaboration is protecting outdoor recreation and a healthy environment. Many Iron Rangers are active outdoorspeople. They want jobs *and* a healthy environment with clean air and water for future generations. Thus, there is potential for environmentalists, Iron Range residents, and unions to unify around ensuring that mining does not pollute water, disrupt wild-game habitat and populations, and limit access to public land. So far, the challenge is in rural-urban and class differences in outdoor-recreation cultures—whether people canoe or use motorboats. Conflicts over conservation and outdoor recreation in northern Minnesota and towns like Ely have simmered for generations; many Iron Rangers *still* view the creation of the BWCAW and wilderness restrictions on motor-vehicle usage as impositions on their rights to use the land. Ultimately, Iron Rangers are the fence-line communities for the proposed copper-nickel mines, and they will endure the immediate effects of air and water pollution whether or not they are directly employed by and risking their health in the mine operations.[29] We can no longer allow corporations to exploit identity conflicts in order to endanger these communities, nor can we ignore the ways those identities have formed and shifted over time. It will be no easy task, but crafting just transitions and more just futures rarely is.

ACKNOWLEDGMENTS

I could not have completed this project without the intellectual, social, logistical, and emotional support from many people along the way. First and foremost, I am grateful to the people in Minnesota who took time to talk with me and welcomed me into their offices, living rooms, and meetings. My research depended on people from environmental groups, government agencies, unions, small businesses, and local government sharing their wisdom and knowledge with me. I appreciate that Ely residents, retired mine workers, and environmental advocates were willing to chat with me and to explain their perspectives and experiences, from which I learned so much.

This book emerged from my research at the University of Minnesota, where I received tremendous support on my intellectual journey. David Pellow, Rachel Schurman, Michael Goldman, and Kate Derickson were vital mentors who pushed me to ask new questions and deepen my analysis while helping me navigate the challenges of fieldwork and data analysis. David has been a wonderfully supportive advisor and collaborator who even in my most uncertain and pessimistic moments gave me confidence and nurtured my ideas. I could always count on Rachel to give incisive edits on drafts and grants proposals. Rachel and Michael also regularly opened their home to lonely and stressed grad students for a warm meal in the dead of Minnesota winter. Other faculty at Minnesota assisted me along the way, including Phyllis Moen, who gave me valuable hands-on research and publishing experience as well as personal support, and Ron Aminzade, who helped me develop the conceptual framing of the project. Debates over Marx and Foucault in Teresa Gowan's living room sparked my intellectual curiosity. I could not have survived completing preliminary exams, conducting fieldwork, and writing a dissertation without my grad-school comrades, especially my cohort members Devika Narayan, Matt Gunther, Jacqui Frost, Erez Garnai, Veronica Horowitz, and Mark Pharris.

I got insightful feedback from many people who read articles, drafts, and proposals and who talked with me over coffee, including Amanda McMillan Lequieu and Ashley Fent. Spending a year as a visiting professor at Davidson College gave me time to work on the manuscript and get feedback from other faculty, including Gerardo Marti, Jennifer Garcia Peacok, and Fuji Lozada. My colleagues at TCU have supported me in pursuing the book, especially our department chair, Carol Thompson, and David Sandel and Dave Aftandilian have given me great advice on the writing and publishing process. Letta Page provided invaluable wordsmithing and helped make the book more coherent, organized, and readable.

My fieldwork was generously funded by the University of Minnesota's College of Liberal Arts Thesis Research Travel Grant and the Department of Sociology's Anna Welsch Bright Research Award. The University of Minnesota Interdisciplinary Doctoral Fellowship enabled me to spend a year writing and collaborating with scholars at the Institute on the Environment. Staff of the University of Minnesota library helped me collect digital data and search the library's archives. Additional funding for transcription, writing, and editing has come from TCU through the Junior Faculty Summer Research Program and the Research and Creative Activities Fund. Participating in the AddRan College Faculty Writing Boot Camp has provided necessary time, structure, and motivation to finish revising the book.

Finally, my partner, Becky, has been with me through thick and thin and given me invaluable social, emotional, and intellectual support. My parents, Shayne and Bill, fostered my passion for workers' rights and the environment and probably never imagined that family stories about northern Minnesota would one day inform a book written by me. My grandparents Rhoda and George Dizard, lifelong union and progressive activists from Duluth, would be dismayed by the current state of politics in Minnesota and the world, but I have hope that their great-grandchild Naomi will experience a more just world.

NOTES

INTRODUCTION

1. Schnaiberg and Gould, *Environment and Society.*
2. Tsing, *Mushroom at the End of the World.*
3. Conde, "Resistance to Mining"; Engels and Dietz, *Contested Extractivism, Society and the State*; Kirsch, *Mining Capitalism*; Schaffartzik et al., "Global Patterns of Metal Extractivism."
4. Alario and Freudenburg, "Paradoxes of Modernity"; Burns, *Bringing down the Mountains*; Finkel and Hays, "Environmental and Health Impacts of 'Fracking'"; Li, *Land's End*; Caruso et al., *Extracting Promises*; Pijpers and Eriksen, *Mining Encounters.*
5. Cramer, *Politics of Resentment*; Hochschild, *Strangers in Their Own Land.*
6. Lipton and Friedman, "Oil Was Central in Decision"; Nash, *Grand Canyon for Sale.*
7. Copper, nickel, and other nonferrous metals (those that do not contain iron) are often found in ore that contains sulfide chemicals. When sulfides are exposed to air and water, sulfuric acid is created, which increases the acidity of water and can leach heavy metals out of surrounding rocks.
8. Bullard, *Dumping in Dixie*; Bullard, "Ecological Inequities and the New South."
9. Gottlieb, *Forcing the Spring*; Taylor, *Rise of the American Conservation Movement.*
10. Freudenburg, "Addictive Economies"; Kazis, Grossman, and Commoner, *Fear at Work*; Beamish, "Environmental Hazard and Institutional Betrayal"; Braun, "Not in My Backyard"; Goodstein, *The Trade-Off Myth*; Matthews, "Enduring Conflict."
11. S. Bell, *Fighting King Coal*; Bell, Fitzgerald, and York, "Protecting the Power to Pollute"; Bell and York, "Community Economic Identity"; Jerolmack and Walker, "Please in My Backyard"; Lewin, "Coal Is Not Just a Job"; Scott, *Removing Mountains.*
12. Andrews and McCarthy, "Scale, Shale, and the State"; Besek, "On the Interactive Nature of Place-Making"; Ferry and Limbert, *Timely Assets*; Wheeler, "Mining Memories in a Rural Community"; Tsing, *Friction.*
13. Manuel, *Taconite Dreams.*
14. Manuel.
15. Marcotty, "Before Copper Pit Opens."
16. Matich, "Look at Historical Copper Prices."
17. Marcotty, "PolyMet Clears a Hurdle."
18. Rootes, "Acting Locally."

19. Casey, *Getting Back into Place*; Escobar, "Culture Sits in Places"; Massey, "Global Sense of Place"; Peck and Yeung, *Remaking the Global Economy*; Sassen, *Globalization and Its Discontents.*
20. S. Bell, *Fighting King Coal*; Marley, "Coal Crisis in Appalachia"; Rolston, *Mining Coal and Undermining Gender.*
21. Freudenburg, "Addictive Economies."
22. Gaventa, *Power and Powerlessness*; Lewin, "Coal Is Not Just a Job"; Scott, "Sociology of Coal Hollow."
23. Landis, *Three Iron Mining Towns*; Manuel, *Taconite Dreams.*
24. Kaunonen, *Flames of Discontent.*
25. Sherman, *Dividing Paradise: Rural Inequality and the Diminishing American Dream*; Abrams and Bliss, "Amenity Landownership"; Farrell, *Billionaire Wilderness.*
26. Manuel, *Taconite Dreams*; Proescholdt, Rapson, and Heinselman, *Troubled Waters.*
27. Norgaard, *Living in Denial.*
28. Boudet et al., "Effect of Industry Activities"; McAdam et al., "Site Fights"; Prudham, *Knock on Wood.*
29. Adams et al., "Forty Years on the Fenceline"; Messer, Shriver, and Adams, "Collective Identity and Memory."
30. Bakker and Bridge, "Material Worlds?"; S. Bell, *Fighting King Coal*; S. Bell, *Our Roots Run Deep as Ironweed*; Bridge, "Contested Terrain"; Gaventa, *Power and Powerlessness*; Hurley and Arı, "Mining (Dis)Amenity"; Malin, *Price of Nuclear Power*; Malin and DeMaster, "Devil's Bargain"; Malin et al., "Right to Resist or a Case of Injustice?"
31. Malin, *Price of Nuclear Power*; Norgaard, *Living in Denial*; Norgaard, "People Want to Protect Themselves."
32. S. Bell, *Fighting King Coal*; Lewin, "Coal Is Not Just a Job"; Shriver, Adams, and Cable, "Discursive Obstruction and Elite Opposition."
33. Johnson, Dowd, and Ridgeway, "Legitimacy as a Social Process."
34. Lamont and Thévenot, *Rethinking Comparative Cultural Sociology*; Sewell, "Theory of Structure."
35. Polletta and Jasper define collective identities as "an individual's cognitive, moral, and emotional connection with a broader community, category, practice, or institution" ("Collective Identity and Social Movements," 285).
36. Gieryn, "Space for Place in Sociology"; Lefebvre, *Production of Space*; Massey, *Space, Place, and Gender*; Soja, *Postmodern Geographies.*
37. Olick, *Collective Memory Reader*; Olick, "Collective Memory"; Zerubavel, *Time Maps.*
38. Polletta and Jasper, "Collective Identity and Social Movements."
39. Wuthnow, *Left Behind.*
40. Bell and York, "Community Economic Identity."
41. Black feminist scholars like Kimberlé Crenshaw, Patricia Hill Collins, and bell hooks developed theories of intersectionality to interrogate the compounding

ways that systems of oppression overlap. Their work emphasized the experiences of Black and other racialized women but is also productive for examining how social class is intertwined with other systems of hierarchy. See Crenshaw, "Demarginalizing the Intersection of Race and Sex"; Crenshaw, "Mapping the Margins"; hooks, *Ain't I a Woman*; Collins, *Black Feminist Thought*; Collins, "Toward a New Vision."

42. I am interested in how my participants understand class in ways that might not fit theoretical definitions or objective measures—particularly how the language of class serves as a code for rural-urban divisions, whiteness, and masculinity. I use the term "working class" to describe an identity as well as a social location and power relationship. Being working class means in part working for a wage, often doing physical labor in industrial and service jobs, having little authority within workplace hierarchies, and typically having less formal education. Being working class is also an identity shaped by people's cultural milieus and habitus, including place, family histories, and types of outdoor recreation. Thus, a fifty-year-old mine worker who never attended college is working class even though he could make more than a retired public school teacher from the Minneapolis suburbs who relocated to Ely. I also distinguish working-class from middle-class people, who are typically professionals in white-collar jobs who have college educations, more authority and autonomy at work, and often, but not always, higher pay and benefits. Being middle class is shaped by cultural tastes, social networks, and where one lives, which, in my study, typically means living in suburbs or cities.
43. Bourdieu, "Social Space and Symbolic Power"; Bourdieu, *Reproduction in Education, Society and Culture*; Thompson, *Making of the English Working Class*; Wacquant, "Making Class."
44. Wealth, education, workplace authority, and social networks provide economic and social capital, while cultural capital consists of tastes, daily habits, hobbies, and language that connotate different levels of social prestige.
45. Bourdieu, *Reproduction in Education, Society and Culture.*
46. Gosnell and Abrams, "Amenity Migration"; Ulrich-Schad and Duncan, "People and Places Left Behind"; Walker and Fortmann, "Whose Landscape?"; R. White, "Are You an Environmentalist?"
47. Whiteness is a constructed racial category used to create systems of hierarchy and to divide poor and working-class people along racial lines. Cheryl Harris describes it as a form of property that is protected and defended. See Roediger, *Wages of Whiteness*; Lipsitz, *Possessive Investment in Whiteness*; Harris, "Whiteness as Property."
48. Roediger, "What If Labor Were Not White and Male?"
49. Roediger, *Wages of Whiteness*; Roediger, "What If Labor Were Not White and Male?"; Mills, "Limitations to Inclusive Unions"; Paap, "How Good Men of the Union Justify Inequality."
50. Filteau, "Who Are Those Guys?"; McHenry, "Getting Fracked"; Scott, "Dependent Masculinity and Political Culture."

51. Western society has associated masculinity with civilization, modernity, and science, while femininity is associated with nature, emotion, and irrationality. See Merchant, *Death of Nature*; Gaard, *Ecofeminism*; Plumwood, *Feminism and the Mastery of Nature*.
52. Masculinities encompass the values, language, practices, roles, and relationships that constitute what it means to be a man in a society. As R. W. Connell theorized, masculinities are socially constructed and variable across time, place, and social location and exist within culture and institutions, including workplaces, rural towns, and organizations—the places where struggles over copper-nickel mining are playing out. Hegemonic masculinity is the idealized form of masculinity that reproduces gender inequality and domination of women while creating a hierarchy of masculinities. See Connell, "Whole New World."
53. Inwood and Bonds, "Property and Whiteness."
54. Daggett, "Petro-Masculinity."
55. Hultman, "Making of an Environmental Hero"; Dockstader and Bell, "Ecomodern Masculinity."
56. There is an extensive literature in environmental history and humanities, and ecofeminism on the meaning of wilderness and nature that explores the linkages between settler colonialism, whiteness, and masculinity. The sociologist Dorceta Taylor has traced the connections between early American environmental thought and conservation leaders with racism, including eugenics, classism, and sexism. See Taylor, *Rise of the American Conservation Movement*.
57. MacGregor, "Stranger Silence Still."
58. Cronon, "Trouble with Wilderness."
59. Connell, "Whole New World."
60. Polletta and Jasper, "Collective Identity and Social Movements"; Goodwin, Jasper, and Polletta, *Passionate Politics*; Jasper, *Art of Moral Protest*; Messer, Shriver, and Adams, "Collective Identity and Memory"; Melucci, "New Social Movements."
61. Benford and Snow, "Framing Processes and Social Movements"; Snow et al., "Frame Alignment Processes."
62. Larsen, "Place Identity"; Mah, *Industrial Ruination*; Norgaard, *Living in Denial*.
63. Bullard, *Dumping in Dixie*; McGurty, *Transforming Environmentalism*; Inwood and Bonds, "Property and Whiteness"; McCarthy, "First World Political Ecology."
64. Gaventa, *Power and Powerlessness*; Bell and York, "Community Economic Identity"; Lewin, "Coal Is Not Just a Job"; Scott, *Removing Mountains*.
65. Dokshin and Buday, "Not in Your Backyard!"; Eaton and Kinchy, "Quiet Voices in the Fracking Debate"; Junod et al., "Life in the Goldilocks Zone"; Kreye, Pienaar, and Adams, "Role of Community Identity"; Ladd, "Environmental Disputes"; Mayer, "Community Economic Identity."
66. Walgrave and Verhulst, "Towards 'New Emotional Movements'?"; Goodwin and Jasper, *Rethinking Social Movements*; Davidson, "Emotion, Reflexivity and Social Change"; Woods et al., "The Country(side) Is Angry"; Norgaard, "'People Want

to Protect Themselves a Little Bit'"; Goodwin, Jasper, and Polletta, *Passionate Politics*; Jacobson, "Sociology of Emotions"; Norgaard, *Living in Denial.*

67. Populism has received renewed scholarly, journalistic, and political attention in the past decade, and there is a lively debate about its utility, definition, and history. I am drawing on definitions of populism as a practice and a discursive and stylistic repertoire, rather than a concrete set of policies or a specific typology. See Bonikowski and Gidron, "Populist Style in American Politics"; Bonikowski, "Three Lessons of Contemporary Populism"; Brubaker, "Why Populism?"; Moffitt, *Global Rise of Populism.*
68. Moffitt, *Global Rise of Populism*; Badiou, *What Is a People*; Grattan, *Populism's Power*; Hall, "Popular-Democratic vs Authoritarian Populism."
69. Laclau, *On Populist Reason*; Mudde, *Populist Radical Right Parties in Europe.*
70. Badiou, *What Is a People*; Hall, "Authoritarian Populism"; Green et al., "Brexit Referendum."
71. Sayer, "Moral Economy and Political Economy."
72. Cole and Foster, *From the Ground Up*; McGurty, *Transforming Environmentalism*; Pellow, *What Is Critical Environmental Justice?*; Taylor, *Rise of the American Conservation Movement.*
73. Gest, Reny, and Mayer, "Roots of the Radical Right."
74. Cramer, *Politics of Resentment*; Hochschild, *Strangers in Their Own Land*; M. Davis, "Great God Trump"; Inglehart and Norris, "Trump, Brexit, and the Rise of Populism"; Oliver and Rahn, "Rise of the Trumpenvolk"; Walley, "Trump's Election and the 'White Working Class.'"
75. Satterfield, *Anatomy of a Conflict*; Sherman, *Dividing Paradise*; Grigsby, *Noodlers in Missouri*; Pulido et al., "Environmental Deregulation."
76. Holstein and Gubrium, *Inside Interviewing.*
77. Rossman and Rallis, *Introduction to Qualitative Research.*
78. Gilchrist and Williams, "Key Informant Interviews"; Rossman and Rallis, *Introduction to Qualitative Research.*
79. The majority of interviews were conducted in person (for logistical reasons, nine were conducted by telephone), usually in public places or the interviewees' office. Occasionally, people invited me to their homes, providing more insights into their private lives. To protect interview participants' identities, I do not use their real names, formal titles, or specific organizational affiliations. I try to ensure respondents' anonymity through pseudonyms while maintaining pertinent details (sometimes including age, race, and type of organizational affiliations), though I include real names and affiliations when quoting public statements including from newspapers and social media posts.
80. Earl et al., "Use of Newspaper Data"; Gamson and Modigliani, "Media Discourse and Public Opinion."
81. Donges and Nitschke, "Political Organizations and Their Online Communication"; Mix and Waldo, "Know(ing) Your Power."

82. Scheman, *Shifting Ground*; Foucault, *Archaeology of Knowledge*.
83. Haraway, *Simians, Cyborgs, and Women*; Harding, *Whose Science?*; Hartsock, *Feminist Standpoint Revisited*; Collins, *Black Feminist Thought*.
84. LaDuke, *All Our Relations*; LaDuke and Carlson, *Our Manoomin, Our Life*; Whyte, "Settler Colonialism"; Norgaard, *Salmon and Acorns Feed Our People*; Grossman, *Unlikely Alliances*; Pasternak, *Grounded Authority*; Simpson, *Mohawk Interruptus*; Deloria and Lytle, *Nations Within*; Hoover, *River Is in Us*.

1. A CONTESTED PLACE

1. Minnesota Department of Natural Resources, *Inter-Agency Task Force Report on Base Metal Mining Impacts*.
2. Pellow and Park, *Silicon Valley of Dreams*.
3. Stark, "Marked by Fire"; Treuer, *Ojibwe in Minnesota*.
4. Doerfler and Redix, "Regional and Tribal Histories."
5. Stark, "Respect, Responsibility, and Renewal."
6. Doerfler and Redix, "Regional and Tribal Histories."
7. Stone, "Treaty of La Pointe."
8. Barzen, "Minnesota Forestry History Stories."
9. E. White, *2017 Regional Profile*.
10. Lamppa, *Minnesota's Iron Country*.
11. Manuel, "Efficiency, Economics, and Environmentalism"; Manuel, *Taconite Dreams*; Lamppa, *Minnesota's Iron Country*.
12. Lamppa, *Minnesota's Iron Country*.
13. Manuel, *Taconite Dreams*.
14. Manuel.
15. Manuel.
16. Lamppa, *Minnesota's Iron Country*.
17. Manuel, *Taconite Dreams*.
18. Manuel, "Efficiency, Economics, and Environmentalism."
19. Manuel.
20. Manuel, *Taconite Dreams*.
21. Lamppa, *Minnesota's Iron Country*.
22. Manuel, *Taconite Dreams*.
23. Lamppa, *Minnesota's Iron Country*.
24. Eleff, "1916 Minnesota Miners' Strike."
25. Lamppa, *Minnesota's Iron Country*.
26. Manuel, *Taconite Dreams*.
27. Lamppa, *Minnesota's Iron Country*.
28. Sherman, *Dividing Paradise*; Sherman, "Coping with Rural Poverty."
29. Nemanic, *One Day for Democracy*.
30. Erlandson, "Why Is Minnesota's Democratic Party Called the DFL?"
31. Brown, *Overburden*, 184.
32. Nemanic, *One Day for Democracy*.

33. Brown, *Overburden*, 45.
34. Brown, *Overburden*.
35. Nemanic, *One Day for Democracy*.
36. Backes, *Canoe Country*.
37. Brown, *Overburden*, 6.
38. Backes, *Canoe Country*.
39. Hemphill, "Explaining the Iron Range Character."
40. Data from US Census Bureau, Annual Community Survey (ACS) 2012–2016 for the Iron Range Resources & Rehabilitation Service Area. Accessed at Wilder Research, "Location Profiles: Iron Range."
41. Waters, *Ethnic Options*.
42. Norrgard, *Seasons of Change*.
43. Parshley, "9 Places to Go to Enjoy the Great Outdoors."
44. Ulrich-Schad and Hua, "Culture Clash?"; Boucquey, "That's My Livelihood"; Nelson, "Rural Restructuring in the American West."
45. Backes, *Canoe Country*.
46. Kess, *More than Just Ore*.
47. Backes, *Canoe Country*; Proescholdt, Rapson, and Heinselman, *Troubled Waters*.
48. Farrell, *Battle for Yellowstone*; Ladino, "Longing for Wonderland"; Malin, *Price of Nuclear Power*; Walker and Fortmann, "Whose Landscape?"
49. Nelson, "Rural Restructuring in the American West"; Ghose, "Big Sky or Big Sprawl?"
50. Adelman, Heberlein, and Bonnicksen, "Social Psychological Explanations"; Jacob and Schreyer, "Conflict in Outdoor Recreation"; Albritton, Stein, and Thapa, "Exploring Conflict and Tolerance."
51. Backes, *Canoe Country*.
52. Proescholdt, Rapson, and Heinselman, *Troubled Waters*.
53. Proescholdt, Rapson, and Heinselman.
54. Backes, *Canoe Country*.
55. Kelleher, "Boundary Waters"; Searle, *Saving Quetico-Superior*.
56. Proescholdt, Rapson, and Heinselman, *Troubled Waters*.
57. Proescholdt, Rapson, and Heinselman, 164.
58. Bierschbach, "How the Specter of the Decades-Long Fight."
59. Proescholdt, Rapson, and Heinselman, *Troubled Waters*.
60. Kennedy, "Looming End of Motorboats Lottery"; Marcotty, "Cell Tower near BWCA Gets OK."
61. Adelman, Heberlein, and Bonnicksen, "Social Psychological Explanations"; Backes, *Canoe Country*.
62. Norrgard, *Seasons of Change*.
63. Child, "Absence of Indigenous Histories."
64. Backes, *Canoe Country*.
65. Chapin, "Challenge to Conservationists"; Dowie, *Conservation Refugees*.
66. Freedman, "When Indigenous Rights and Wilderness Collide."

67. Loew and Thannum, "After the Storm"; Nesper, *Walleye War*.
68. Nesper, *Walleye War*.

2. ACCEPTANCE AND RESISTANCE

1. Marcotty, "Mine's Risks Spotlighted."
2. Feagin, "Extractive Regions in Developed Countries"; Freudenburg, "Addictive Economies"; Freudenburg and Gramling, "Linked to What?"; Frickel and Freudenburg, "Mining the Past."
3. Deloria and Lytle, *Nations Within*; Ali, *Mining, the Environment, and Indigenous Development Conflicts*; Clark, "Indigenous Environmental Movement"; Spice, "Fighting Invasive Infrastructures"; Voyles, *Wastelanding*.
4. Freudenburg, "Addictive Economies"; Widick, *Trouble in the Forest*; Lewis, "Appalachian Restructuring in Historical Perspective"; Lobao et al., "Poverty, Place, and Coal Employment"; Marley, "The Coal Crisis in Appalachia"; Loomis, *Empire of Timber*.
5. Data for West Virginia is from the Appalachian Regional Commission (ARC) compiled by Fahe ("Appalachian Poverty"). Data for Minnesota is from the US Census Bureau, Annual Community Survey (ACS) 2012–2016 for the Iron Range Resources & Rehabilitation Service Area. Accessed at Wilder Research, "Location Profiles: Iron Range."
6. Manuel, *Taconite Dreams*.
7. For St. Louis County, unemployment was 4.5 percent in July 2017, compared to 3.7 percent for the state at large. The Iron Range region also has a lower median income than does the state at large. For example, in 2015, it was $47,564, compared to $67,019 for all of Minnesota. Data for the Iron Range are from the Minnesota Department of Employment and Economic Development, E. White, *2017 Regional Profile*. Statewide and county data are from US Census Bureau, "2013–2017 American Community Survey."
8. E. White, *2017 Regional Profile*.
9. Kraker, "Mine Layoffs."
10. Data for the Minnesota Economic Development Regions, EDR 3–Arrowhead, which encompasses the Iron Range and broader northeastern Minnesota, in 2019. Minnesota Department of Employment and Economic Development, "Quarterly Employment Demographics."
11. Data for the Minnesota Economic Development Regions, EDR 3–Arrowhead. Minnesota Department of Employment and Economic Development.
12. Explore Minnesota, "Tourism and Minnesota's Economy."
13. The median wage in 2019 for jobs in hospitality and food service was $12.01 and for jobs in health care and social services was $19.29. Data from the Minnesota Department of Employment and Economic Development, "Occupational Employment and Wage Statistics," based on quarterly employment demographics for the Arrowhead Economic Development Region.
14. Center for Rural Policy and Development, *State of Rural Minnesota Report 2017*.

15. The median age was fifty years in Ely and forty-five in the Iron Range, compared to the national median age of forty years. Wilder Research, "Location Profiles: Ely"; Wilder Research, "Location Profiles: Iron Range."
16. Wilder Research, "Location Profiles: Iron Range."
17. Manuel, *Taconite Dreams*.
18. St. George, "Long-Range Issue."
19. This type of mining is often called "hardrock mining" to distinguish it from coal, sand, and salt mining. However, I use the term "copper-nickel mining" to emphasize the key metals and to differentiate these nonferrous metals from iron mining, which is also considered hardrock mining. The term "copper-nickel mining" is also more descriptive and less technical than "nonferrous-metal mining."
20. Carter, *Boom, Bust, Boom*; LeCain, *Mass Destruction*; Martinez-Alier, "Mining Conflicts, Environmental Justice, and Valuation."
21. Carter, *Boom, Bust, Boom*; LeCain, *Mass Destruction*.
22. Brininstool and Flanagan, "2015 Minerals Yearbook"; G. Ross, "Copper, Nickel, Lead & Zinc Mining."
23. G. Ross, "Copper, Nickel, Lead & Zinc Mining."
24. Guyer, "Oil Assemblages and the Production of Confusion."
25. Arboleda, "Financialization, Totality and Planetary Urbanization"; Labban, "Oil in Parallax."
26. Investing News Network, "10 Top Copper-Producing Companies"; DePass, "Revival on the Range."
27. G. Ross, "Copper, Nickel, Lead & Zinc Mining."
28. Matich, "Look at Historical Copper Prices."
29. Pantland, "Glencore."
30. Kneas, "Subsoil Abundance and Surface Absence."
31. Arboleda, "Financialization, Totality and Planetary Urbanization"; Bunker and Ciccantell, *Globalization and the Race for Resources*.
32. Investing News Network, "10 Top Copper-Producing Companies."
33. Scheyder and Lewis, "Glencore's Risk Appetite Dwindles."
34. Gestring, *U.S. Copper Porphyry Mines Report*.
35. Earthworks, "Financial Assurance and Superfund"; US Government Accountability Office, "Environmental Liabilities."
36. Guarino, "Thousands of Montana Snow Geese Die."
37. Martinez-Alier, "Mining Conflicts, Environmental Justice, and Valuation."
38. Gestring, *U.S. Copper Porphyry Mines Report*; Jacobs, Testa, and Lehr, *Acid Mine Drainage*.
39. Fruehan, *Making, Shaping, and Treating of Steel*; Lapakko, "Prediction of Acid Mine Drainage"; Onello et al., "Sulfide Mining and Human Health."
40. Minnesota Environmental Quality Board, *Minnesota Regional Copper-Nickel Study*.
41. Minnesota Department of Natural Resources, US Army Corps of Engineers, and US Forest Service, "Factsheet."

42. Onello et al., "Sulfide Mining and Human Health."
43. Minnesota Department of Natural Resources, US Army Corps of Engineers, and US Forest Service, "Factsheet."
44. Researchers found that runoff from test-sample ores from the Duluth Complex are capable of generating acid mine drainage, and analysis by independent scientists reveals that runoff would probably exceed water-quality standards and contain heavy metals. See L. Anderson, "Copper-Nickel Controversy"; Center for Science in Public Participation, *Potential for Acid Mine Drainage*; Lapakko, Olson, and Antonson, *Dissolution of Duluth Complex Rock*.
45. Lapakko and Antonson, *Duluth Complex Rock Dissolution and Mitigation Techniques*"; Minnesota Environmental Quality Board, *Minnesota Regional Copper-Nickel Study*.
46. Author interview with Dan Jones, professor of geobiology at University of Minnesota, May 11, 2017.
47. Schuldt et al., "Expanding the Narrative of Tribal Health."
48. Schuldt et al.; Myrbo et al., "Sulfide Generated by Sulfate Reduction"; Moyle, "Some Chemical Factors."
49. Coleman, "Iron Mining in Minnesota."
50. Onello et al., "Sulfide Mining and Human Health"; World Health Organization, "Mercury and Health."
51. Fetal brain development may be impacted by exposure to mercury. For an overview of the health risks and warning, see Minnesota Department of Health, "Minnesota Fish."
52. Kojola, "Indigeneity, Gender, and Class."
53. Davies, "Tailings Impoundment Failures"
54. Minnesota Center for Environmental Advocacy, "Protecting Minnesota."
55. With dry stacking, the leftover rock is piled up and covered in soil and vegetation, preventing exposure to air and water and thus eliminating the risks of maintaining ponds and dams.
56. Bjorhus, "Mine Promises No Acid Drainage."
57. Marcotty, "Mine Review Delayed Again"; Minnesota Department of Natural Resources, US Army Corps of Engineers, and US Forest Service, "Factsheet."
58. Kuipers et al., *Comparison of Predicted and Actual Water Quality*.
59. Center for Science in Public Participation, *Potential for Acid Mine Drainage*; Conservation Minnesota, Friends of the Boundary Waters Wilderness, Minnesota Center for Environmental Advocacy, "Frequently Asked Questions."
60. Center for Science in Public Participation, *Potential for Acid Mine Drainage*.
61. Gestring, *U.S. Copper Porphyry Mines Report*; Kuipers et al., *Comparison of Predicted and Actual Water Quality*.
62. Davies, "Tailings Impoundment Failures"; Minnesota Department of Health, *Minnesota Climate and Health Profile Report 2015*.
63. T. Myers, *Technical Memorandum*.

64. In the flotation process, the ore is crushed into a powder and mixed with water to create a slurry that is suspended in liquid in order to separate out the valuable metals. The resulting concentrate is then refined into a marketable product through additional techniques, such as smelting or hydrometallurgy, that can be done on- or off-site.
65. Onello et al., "Sulfide Mining and Human Health."
66. Asbestos-like fibers impact the human respiratory system and can cause lung cancer.
67. Onello et al., "Sulfide Mining and Human Health."
68. Minnesota Department of Natural Resources, "State Nonferrous Metallic Mineral Leasing Purposes and Policies."
69. Raster and Hill, "Dispute over Wild Rice"; LaDuke and Carlson, *Our Manoomin, Our Life*.
70. Doerfler and Redix, "Regional and Tribal Histories."
71. Estes, *Our History Is the Future*; Gedicks, *New Resource Wars*; Grossman, *Unlikely Alliances*.
72. Estes, *Our History Is the Future*; Nesper, *Walleye War*; Norrgard, *Seasons of Change*; Raster and Hill, "Dispute over Wild Rice"; Loew and Thannum, "After the Storm"; Stark, "Respect, Responsibility, and Renewal"; Stark, "Marked by Fire"; Allison, *Sovereignty for Survival*; Moreton-Robinson, *White Possessive*; Pasternak, *Grounded Authority*; L. Simpson, *As We Have Always Done*.
73. Voyles, *Wastelanding*.
74. Minnesota Environmental Quality Board, *Minnesota Regional Copper-Nickel Study*.
75. L. Anderson, "Copper-Nickel Controversy."
76. The final report concluded that mining could be done within environmental regulations but nonetheless involved serious social and environmental risks. Minnesota Environmental Quality Board, *Minnesota Regional Copper-Nickel Study*.
77. Rebuffoni, "Kennecott to Take Over Stalled Copper Project."
78. The plan projects eighteen months for construction and a twenty-year operation horizon, with production estimates at 72 million pounds of copper, 15.4 million pounds of nickel, and 720,000 pounds of cobalt and other metals through the removal of 533 million tons of ore and waste rock. Project details come from Minnesota Department of Natural Resources, US Army Corps of Engineers, and US Forest Service, "Final Environmental Impact Statement—Appendix C."
79. In Minnesota and much of the western US, the subsurface mineral rights can be owned separately from the surface land rights in what is called a "split-estate."
80. Minnesota Department of Natural Resources, US Army Corps of Engineers, and US Forest Service, "Final Environmental Impact Statement."
81. Conservation Minnesota, Friends of the Boundary Waters Wilderness, and Minnesota Center for Environmental Advocacy, "Frequently Asked Questions."
82. Oakes, "North Country Blues"; J. Ross, "Another Small-Town Minnesota Grocery Store."

83. Bloomquist, "Company Still Hopes"; FTSE Russell, "Company Report."
84. Orenstein, "PolyMet Is Now Owned by Switzerland's Glencore."
85. Ramstad, "PolyMet Receives $14 Million."
86. Minnesota Department of Natural Resources, US Army Corps of Engineers, and US Forest Service, "Final Environmental Impact Statement—Appendix C."
87. Fond du Lac Band of Lake Superior Chippewa, "Complaint for Declaratory and Injunctive Relief."
88. Fond du Lac Band of Lake Superior Chippewa, "Ojibwe Place Names."
89. Conservation Minnesota, Friends of the Boundary Waters Wilderness, Minnesota Center for Environmental Advocacy, "Frequently Asked Questions."
90. Fond du Lac Band of Lake Superior Chippewa, "Complaint for Declaratory and Injunctive Relief."
91. Minnesota Department of Natural Resources, US Army Corps of Engineers, and US Forest Service, "Final Environmental Impact Statement."
92. Minnesota Department of Natural Resources, US Army Corps of Engineers, and US Forest Service, "Final Environmental Impact Statement—Appendix C," 4-340.
93. An EIS involves evaluating the potential environmental impacts, assessing alternatives, and developing plans for mitigation after operation. The PolyMet EIS was triggered by the National Environmental Policy Act (NEPA) and the Minnesota Environmental Protection Act (MEPA). Initially, the EIS process was led by the US Army Corps of Engineers, which oversees all development impacting waterways and wetlands. US Environmental Protection Agency, "National Environmental Policy Act Review Process."
94. "Metals Mining Company Begins."
95. J. Myers, "PolyMet, Environmentalists Square Off."
96. The EPA cited a lack of detail, criticized the data used in the analysis for water-pollution models, voiced concerns about the serious risks of acid mine drainage and the loss of thousands of acres of federal land and wetlands, and raised doubts about the company's financial assurances to fund future cleanup costs. Shaffer, "PolyMet Committed to Disputed Mine Plan."
97. Research in California found that over a twenty-three-year period, the EPA regional office only deemed about four in three thousand EISs "unsatisfactory." Simons, "Mining Face-Off."
98. Shaffer, "PolyMet Committed to Disputed Mine Plan."
99. Shaffer, "PolyMet Mining Hires Former MPCA Commissioner."
100. Shaffer, "PolyMet Committed."
101. Meersman, "Proposed Copper-Nickel Mine."
102. Marcotty, "Battle Waged over Mining Firms' Plans."
103. J. Myers, "Anti-Mining Rally Targets Duluth Chamber."
104. Jobs for Minnesotans, "About Us."
105. "No Extra Mine Comment Time."
106. Marcotty, "PolyMet Copper Mine."
107. Marcotty, "PolyMet Clears a Hurdle."

108. Mitchell, "Minnesota Poll."
109. J. Myers, "Critics' Poll Shows Growing Opposition."
110. In December 2017, PolyMet offered just $65 million in credit or bonds and $10 million in cash to cover liabilities during construction. But according to the initial estimates, that amount would expand to $544 million once the mine is in operation. Helmberger, "PolyMet Adds More Money."
111. Helmberger, "PolyMet's Financial Prospects Dim."
112. Bjorhus, "Copper Mine Leases Denied"; Twin Metals Minnesota, "About the Project."
113. Bjorhus, "Mine Promises No Acid Drainage."
114. Twin Metals was incorporated in Canada in January 2010 as a partnership between Duluth Metals Limited and the Chilean Antofagasta PLC. In 2015, Antofagasta bought Duluth Metals, making Twin Metals a subsidiary of the Chilean company. See Shaffer, "Range Copper Firms"; Twin Metals Minnesota, "About the Project."
115. Bjorhus, "Mine Promises No Acid Drainage"; St. Anthony, "Officials Tout Benefits of Mine."
116. J. Myers, "Fed Shutdown Delays Review."
117. Minnesota Environmental Quality Board, *Minnesota Regional Copper-Nickel Study*.
118. The Twin Metals proposal also includes a plan to backfill the underground mine when operations stop, with some of the tailings and waste rock kept in dry-stack storage. See Bjorhus, "Mine Promises No Acid Drainage"; Twin Metals Minnesota, "About the Project."
119. Frelich, "Forest and Terrestrial Ecosystem Impacts."
120. Minnesota Department of Natural Resources, US Army Corps of Engineers, and US Forest Service, "NorthMet Mining Project."
121. Backes, *Canoe Country*.
122. Wilder Research, "Location Profiles: Ely"; Wilder Research, "Minnesota's Population."
123. Ely's median household income was $35,288 in 2016, compared to the state's median income of $67,867. US Census Bureau, "2013–2017 American Community Survey."
124. US Census Bureau, "2011–2015 American Community Survey."
125. In 2015, the median family income in Ely was $36,059, compared to $54,022 in nearby Morse Township or $62,500 in Fall Lake Township, where many of the new residents live. US Census Bureau.
126. Data from Office of Minnesota Secretary of State, "2016 General Election Results."
127. Campaign to Save the Boundary Waters, "Timeline."
128. Campaign to Save the Boundary Waters, "About the Campaign."
129. Ode, "Testing Their Boundary"; Freeman and Freeman, *Year in the Wilderness*.
130. Drucker, "More than 200 Businesses Join Forces."
131. Anzalone Liszt Grove Research, "Summary of Registered Voters"; Anzalone Liszt Grove Research, "Minnesotans Strongly Oppose."

132. J. Myers, "Dayton Calls Twin Metals Mine a Threat."
133. Marcotty, "Dayton Rebuffs Twin Metals Mine Proposal."
134. Such leases typically have a finite length and must be renewed by the US Bureau of Land Management and US Forest Service. Bjorhus, "Copper Mine Leases Denied."
135. Marcotty, "Agency Airs Concerns."
136. Mouritsen, "Decision."
137. Bjorhus, "Copper Mine Leases Denied."
138. This is the longest ban the secretary of the interior could implement without an act of Congress.
139. J. Myers, "Twin Metals Gets Federal Mining Leases Back."
140. Brooks, "Forest Service Scales Back Environmental Study."
141. The data and analysis initially conducted for the EA have not been publicly released, though environmentalists, Democratic politicians, and media outlets are vigorously demanding that the information be shared. See Bjorhus, "McCollum Fighting for Mine Study."
142. Tobias, "Meet the Former Koch Adviser."
143. Friends of the Boundary Waters Wilderness, "How Cozy Is Twin Metals with the Trump Administration?"
144. Whieldon and Snider, "Trump's Interior Pick Lifts Outdoors Groups."
145. Lipton and Friedman, "Oil Was Central in Decision to Shrink Bears Ears Monument, Emails Show."
146. Tabuchi, "Biden Administration Cancels Mining Leases."
147. "Minnesota DNR Stops Work."
148. There is some debate about whether water from the PolyMet site could enter the BWCAW. Analysis by scientists for the Great Lakes Indian Fish and Wildlife Commission found that water could flow northward toward the BWCAW. This contradicts water modeling conducted by state and federal agencies. The agencies responded by saying the northward flow was unlikely but a "theoretical possibility" and said they would investigate. See Dunbar, "Alleged Risk to BWCA."
149. Baker, "Potential Ecological Impacts"; Minnesota Environmental Quality Board, *Minnesota Regional Copper-Nickel Study*.

3. KNOWING THE LAND

1. Eliasoph and Lichterman, "Culture in Interaction."
2. Voyles, *Wastelanding*.
3. MacGregor, "Stranger Silence Still."
4. Bullard, *Dumping in Dixie*; Cole and Foster, *From the Ground Up*; Mohai, Pellow, and Roberts, "Environmental Justice"; Sze, *Noxious New York*; Szasz, *Ecopopulism*.
5. Dear, "Understanding and Overcoming the NIMBY Syndrome"; Devine-Wright, "Rethinking NIMBYism"; Larson and Krannich, "Great Idea"; Phadke, "Resisting and Reconciling Big Wind."
6. Escobar, "Culture Sits in Places."

7. Boudet et al., "Effect of Industry Activities"; Clarke et al., "How Geographic Distance and Political Ideology Interact"; Dokshin, "Whose Backyard and What's at Issue?"; Gravelle and Lachapelle, "Politics, Proximity and the Pipeline"; Mix and Waldo, "Know(ing) Your Power."
8. Daggett, "Petro-Masculinity."
9. Scott, *Removing Mountains*.
10. Minnesota Department of Employment and Economic Development, "Occupational Employment and Wage Statistics."
11. Mishkind, "Sexual Harassment Hostile Work Environment Class Actions."
12. Wuthnow, *Left Behind*.
13. Threadgold et al., "Affect, Risk and Local Politics of Knowledge"; Wheeler, "Mining Memories in a Rural Community"; Wheeler, "Local History as Productive Nostalgia?"
14. Meier, "Metalworkers' Nostalgic Memories."
15. Massey, *Space, Place, and Gender*; McAdam and Boudet, *Putting Social Movements in Their Place*.
16. Messer, Shriver, and Adams, "Collective Identity and Memory"; Neumann, "Toxic Talk and Collective (In)Action in a Company Town"; Kreye, Pienaar, and Adams, "Role of Community Identity"; Zavestoski et al., "Toxicity and Complicity."
17. Scott, *Removing Mountains*.
18. Berns and Simpson, "Outdoor Recreation Participation."
19. Farrell, *Battle for Yellowstone*.
20. Taylor, *Rise of the American Conservation Movement*; DeLuca and Demo, "Imagining Nature and Erasing Class and Race"; Brechin, "Conserving the Race."
21. Plumwood, *Feminism and the Mastery of Nature*; Sturgeon, *Ecofeminist Natures*.
22. Norgaard, *Living in Denial*.
23. DeLuca and Demo, "Imagining Nature and Erasing Class and Race."
24. Cronon, "Trouble with Wilderness"; Cronon, *Uncommon Ground*; Spence, *Dispossessing the Wilderness*.
25. R. White, "Are You an Environmentalist?"
26. Moe, "Rushing to Ruin the Boundary Waters Wilderness."
27. Minnesota Pollution Control Agency, "St. Louis River."
28. US Environmental Protection Agency, "About the St. Louis River and Bay AOC."
29. Friends of the Boundary Waters Wilderness, Minnesota Center for Environmental Advocacy, Center for Biological Diversity, and Earth Justice. "Lawsuit Targets Minnesota's PolyMet Copper-Sulfide Mine Permit."
30. Fond du Lac Band of Lake Superior Chippewa, "Complaint for Declaratory and Injunctive Relief."
31. Fond du Lac Band of Lake Superior Chippewa, Grand Portage Band of Lake Superior Chippewa, Bois Forte Band of Chippewa, Great Lakes Indian Fish & Wildlife Commission, and the 1854 Treaty Authority, "How Will Cultural Resources Be Affected by the NorthMet Mine?"
32. Myrbo et al., "Sulfide Generated by Sulfate Reduction."

33. Freedman, "When Indigenous Rights and Wilderness Collide."
34. Barker and Pickerill, "Radicalizing Relationships"; Ranco and Suagee, "Tribal Sovereignty"; Moore, "Coalition Building"; Grossman, *Unlikely Alliances*.
35. Gedicks, *New Resource Wars*; Grossman, *Unlikely Alliances*.
36. WaterLegacy, "Oppose the PolyMet NorthMet Sulfide Mine."
37. Taylor, *Rise of the American Conservation Movement*; Cole and Foster, *From the Ground Up*; Gottlieb, *Forcing the Spring*.
38. Guarino, "Thousands of Montana Snow Geese Die."
39. Grigsby, *Noodlers in Missouri*; Sherman, *Dividing Paradise*.
40. Jacoby, *Crimes against Nature*; R. White, "Are You an Environmentalist?"
41. Desmond, *On the Fireline*; Grigsby, *Noodlers in Missouri*.
42. Satterfield, *Anatomy of a Conflict*.
43. Ashwood, *For-Profit Democracy*.
44. M. Bell, *Childerley*.
45. Bosworth, "'They're Treating Us like Indians!'"
46. Anshelm and Hultman, "Green Fatwā?"
47. Greer and Bruno, *Greenwash*.
48. Phadke, "Green Energy Futures."
49. Bell and York, "Community Economic Identity"; Mix and Waldo, "Know(ing) Your Power."
50. Hobsbawm, "Introduction."
51. Malin, *Price of Nuclear Power*; Malin et al., "Right to Resist or a Case of Injustice?"; Sze et al., "Defining and Contesting Environmental Justice."
52. Malin, *Price of Nuclear Power*.
53. Jones and Garde-Hansen, *Geography and Memory*; Muehlebach, "Body of Solidarity"; Freudenburg, Frickel, and Gramling, "Beyond the Nature/Society Divide."
54. Freudenburg, Frickel, and Gramling, "Beyond the Nature/Society Divide."

4. MINING MEMORIES

1. Baker, Ekstrom, and Bedsworth, "Climate Information?"; Burnham et al., "Politics of Imaginaries"; Mische, "Measuring Futures in Action."
2. Strangleman, "Smokestack Nostalgia."
3. Adam, *Timescapes of Modernity*; J. White, "Climate Change and the Generational Timescape."
4. Olick, *Collective Memory Reader*; Olick and Robbins, "Social Memory Studies"; Kubal and Becerra, "Social Movements and Collective Memory."
5. Massey, "Places and Their Pasts," 186.
6. Olick and Robbins, "Social Memory Studies"; Hodgkin and Radstone, *Contested Pasts*; Lipsitz, *Time Passages*; Molden, "Resistant Pasts versus Mnemonic Hegemony."
7. Fent and Kojola, "Political Ecologies of Time"; Mukta and Hardiman, "The Political Ecology of Nostalgia"; Norgaard, *Living in Denial*; Raynes et al., "Emotional Landscape of Place-Based Activism"; Scott, "Environmental Affects"; Bonnett,

Left in the Past; Campbell, Smith, and Wetherell, "Nostalgia and Heritage"; Smith and Campbell, "Nostalgia for the Future."

8. Bonnett and Alexander, "Mobile Nostalgias"; Boym, *Future of Nostalgia*; F. Davis, *Yearning for Yesterday*; Legg, "Memory and Nostalgia."
9. Bonnett, *Left in the Past*.
10. Blunt, "Collective Memory and Productive Nostalgia"; Boym, *Future of Nostalgia*; Lowenthal, *Past Is a Foreign Country*; Smith and Campbell, "Nostalgia for the Future."
11. Strangleman, "Smokestack Nostalgia."
12. Wheeler, "Mining Memories in a Rural Community."
13. Strangleman, "Smokestack Nostalgia."
14. Allister, introduction to *Eco-Man*.
15. Strangleman, "Smokestack Nostalgia."
16. Roberts, "Collective Representations"; Hodgkin and Radstone, "Introduction."
17. Mathews and Barnes, "Prognosis"; Weszkalnys, "Doubtful Hope."
18. Brown, *Overburden*.
19. PolyMet, "Community and Economic Benefits."
20. Huber, *Lifeblood*; Lewin, "Coal Is Not Just a Job"; Scott, *Removing Mountains*; Rolston, *Mining Coal and Undermining Gender*.
21. Bingham and Gansler, *Class Action*.
22. Connell, "Whole New World."
23. Hodgkin and Radstone, *Contested Pasts*; Jones and Garde-Hansen, *Geography and Memory*; Wheeler, "Mining Memories in a Rural Community."
24. Hodgkin and Radstone, *Contested Pasts*.
25. Manuel, *Taconite Dreams*.
26. Manuel.
27. Manuel.
28. Iron Mining Association of Minnesota, "Role of the IMA."
29. "Now What?"
30. Helmberger, "PolyMet's Financial Prospects Dim"; Helmberger, "Court Hears Arguments."
31. Acharya, Paudel, and Hatch, "Impact of Nostalgia and Past Experience"; Ladino, *Reclaiming Nostalgia*; Ladino, "Longing for Wonderland."
32. Cronon, *Uncommon Ground*.
33. Allister, introduction to *Eco-Man*.
34. Lopez, "Paddler's View."
35. Proescholdt, Rapson, and Heinselman, *Troubled Waters*.
36. Martinez-Alier, "Environmentalism of the Poor"; Taylor, "Women of Color"; Sturgeon, *Ecofeminist Natures*.
37. Finney, *Black Faces, White Spaces*; Taylor, *Rise of the American Conservation Movement*; Barca, "On Working-Class Environmentalism."
38. US Environmental Protection Agency, "Hardrock Mining: Environmental Impacts."

39. Marcotty, "Lawsuit Alleges Lax Regulation."
40. Hana, "PolyMet EIS Takes a Big Step."
41. Bartlett, *Reserve Mining Controversy*.
42. Langston, *Sustaining Lake Superior*.
43. Tomassoni, "Mining Is Us."
44. "Now What?"
45. Rudacille, "How Toxic Is Smokestack Nostalgia?"
46. US Government Accountability Office, "Environmental Liabilities"; US Environmental Protection Agency, "Hardrock Mining"; Carter, *Boom, Bust, Boom*.
47. American Rivers, "America's Most Endangered Rivers 2015."
48. Baeten, Langston, and Lafreniere, "Spatial Evaluation"; Langston, *Sustaining Lake Superior*.
49. Langston, *Sustaining Lake Superior*; Myrbo et al., "Sulfide Generated by Sulfate Reduction"; Baeten, Langston, and Lafreniere, "Spatial Evaluation."
50. Minnesota Department of Health, *Mesothelioma in Northeastern Minnesota*.
51. Finnegan and Mandel, "Final Report to the Legislature."
52. Burnham et al., "Politics of Imaginaries"; Messer, Shriver, and Adams, "Collective Identity and Memory"; Adam, *Timescapes of Modernity*; Mathews and Barnes, "Prognosis."
53. Kneas, "Subsoil Abundance and Surface Absence."
54. Ramirez, "Both Sides Agree."
55. Manuel, *Taconite Dreams*.
56. The University of Minnesota has a long history of conducting research on mining technology and engineering for industry use and in exploration of new deposits.
57. Manuel, *Taconite Dreams*.
58. Lovrien, "Minnesota's Only Solar Panel Manufacturer."
59. Frickel and Freudenburg, "Mining the Past"; Lewin, "Coal Is Not Just a Job"; Wheeler, "Local History as Productive Nostalgia?"
60. Blunt, "Collective Memory and Productive Nostalgia"; Bonnett, *Left in the Past*; Pickering and Keightley, "Modalities of Nostalgia"; Smith and Campbell, "Nostalgia for the Future."
61. Strangleman, "Smokestack Nostalgia"; Rudacille, "How Toxic Is Smokestack Nostalgia?"

5. EXTRACTIVE POPULISM

1. Butler, "Reflections on Trump"; Packer, "Hillary Clinton and the Populist Revolt"; Walley, "Trump's Election and the 'White Working Class.'"
2. Oliver and Rahn, "Rise of the Trumpenvolk."
3. Marcotty, "Dayton Rebuffs Twin Metals Mine Proposal."
4. Burnes, "DFL Considering Resolution 54."
5. Myers, "Emmer, Nolan Add Amendment."

6. The MINER Act passed the US House in 2017 but as of 2022 had not received a vote in the US Senate, and its prospects are uncertain after Democrats took power in 2020. Coombe, "MINER Act Passes House."
7. Bobo, "Racism in Trump's America"; Inglehart and Norris, "Trump, Brexit, and the Rise of Populism."
8. M. Davis, "Great God Trump"; Edsall and Edsall, *Chain Reaction*; Teixeira and Rogers, *America's Forgotten Majority*.
9. Manuel, *Taconite Dreams*.
10. Kraker, "Iron Range Voters Turn to Trump."
11. Data from Office of Minnesota Secretary of State, "2016 General Election Results," for precincts 6A and 6B, which include Hibbing and Virginia, Minnesota.
12. Sherry, "Rick Nolan Wins Again."
13. "Minnesota 2016 Presidential Caucus Results."
14. Huber, *Lifeblood*.
15. Daggett, "Petro-Masculinity"; Scott, "Dependent Masculinity and Political Culture."
16. Boucquey, "That's My Livelihood"; McCarthy, "First World Political Ecology."
17. Haney-López, *Dog Whistle Politics*; Niemonen, "Emotional Politics of Racism"; C. Anderson, *White Rage*; Bonilla-Silva, *Racism without Racists*; Lipsitz, *Possessive Investment in Whiteness*.
18. Scoones et al., "Emancipatory Rural Politics"; Holloway, "Burning Issues."
19. Wuthnow, *Left Behind*.
20. Manuel, *Taconite Dreams*.
21. Backes, *Canoe Country*; Manuel, *Taconite Dreams*.
22. US Census Bureau, "2013–2017 American Community Survey."
23. Office of Minnesota Secretary of State, "2016 General Election Results."
24. Malin, *Price of Nuclear Power*; Shumway and Jackson, "Place Making"; Ulrich-Schad and Hua, "Culture Clash?"
25. Bourdieu, *Reproduction in Education*.
26. Rowell, *Green Backlash*; Turner, "Specter of Environmentalism."
27. Kojola, "(Re)constructing the Pipeline."
28. Arvin, "Indigenous-Led Fight."
29. Tyler, "Time for Anti-Mining Accountability."
30. Montrie, *Making a Living*; Gottlieb, *Forcing the Spring*.
31. Forgrave, "In Northern Minnesota, Two Economies Square Off."
32. Foster, "Limits of Environmentalism without Class"; Loomis, *Empire of Timber*; Rose, *Coalitions across the Class Divide*.
33. Nolan, "Nolan Brings Down the Hammer."
34. Sheridan, "Embattled Ranchers"; Robbins et al., "Writing the New West."
35. Hochschild, *Strangers in Their Own Land*.
36. Wuthnow, *Left Behind*.
37. Chezick, "Let's Help the Anti-Mining Dems Lose."
38. Scoones et al., "Emancipatory Rural Politics"; Holloway, "Burning Issues."

39. Arbatli, "Resource Nationalism Revisited"; Bridge, "Resource Geographies II"; Kohl and Farthing, "Material Constraints to Popular Imaginaries."
40. Smith, *National Identity*; Taggart, *Populism*.
41. Natural Resource Research Institute, "NRRI Geologists Define Minnesota Resources."
42. Adams and Glück, "Financialization in Commodity Markets"; G. Davis, *Managed by the Markets*; Labban, "Oil in Parallax."
43. Steine, "Thoughts on Mining's Past."
44. US Geological Survey, *Mineral Commodity Summaries 2018*.
45. Simoes, "Copper Ore"; Simoes, "Nickel Ore."
46. Marcotty, "Minnesota's Mining Boom"; Rivera, "Copper Is Up on a Six-Month High."
47. Mui, "Financial Turmoil Half a World Away."
48. Myers, "PolyMet Will Trade More Stock for Cash."
49. Brodey, "Is Steel Dumping the Real Culprit?"
50. Coolican, "Politicians Try to Bring Aid"; DePass, "New Trade Tariffs Thwart Steel Dumping"; Myers, "Keetac to Reopen."
51. Nolan, "Nolan Brings Down the Hammer."
52. Turkewitz, "Bundy Brothers Defend Armed Occupation."
53. Bennett, *Logic of Connective Action*; Kidd and McIntosh, "Social Media and Social Movements."
54. Tobias, "Meet the Former Koch Adviser."
55. Helgeson, "Mine Project Tests DFL Unity."
56. Sherry, "Eighth Congressional District."
57. Pliml, "Despite Concerns, Staying Blue."
58. Ramirez, "Both Sides Agree."
59. Behsudi, "Minnesota on the Edge"
60. Prescod, "We Can't Abandon the Building Trades Unions."
61. "Glencore, Steelworkers in Sudbury, Reach Deal"; Bronfrenbrenner and Juravich, "Evolution of Strategic and Coordinated Bargaining Campaigns"; Dewey, "Working for the Environment."
62. Onello et al., "Sulfide Mining and Human Health."
63. Brecher and Labor Network for Sustainability, "Stormy Weather"; Stevis, "Deep Cleavages"; Sweeney, "Contested Futures."
64. Taggart, *Populism*.
65. Scoones et al., "Emancipatory Rural Politics."
66. Gusterson, "From Brexit to Trump"; Skocpol, *Tea Party*; Walley, "Trump's Election and the 'White Working Class.'"
67. Frank, *Listen, Liberal*; McQuarrie, "Revolt of the Rust Belt."

CONCLUSION

1. Sherman, *Dividing Paradise*; Ghose, "Big Sky or Big Sprawl?"; Ulrich-Schad and Hua, "Culture Clash?"
2. Kazis, Grossman, and Commoner, *Fear at Work*.

3. Norgaard, *Living in Denial*; Norgaard and Reed, "Emotional Impacts of Environmental Decline"; Norgaard, "Climate Denial and the Construction of Innocence."
4. Freudenburg, Frickel, and Gramling, "Beyond the Nature/Society Divide."
5. Jacoby, *Crimes against Nature*; Farrell, *Billionaire Wilderness*; Watt, *Paradox of Preservation*; Cronon, "Trouble with Wilderness."
6. Edsall and Edsall, *Chain Reaction*; Frank, *Listen, Liberal*; Harvey, *Brief History of Neoliberalism*.
7. Morgan and Lee, "Trump Voters and the White Working Class"; Morgan and Lee, "Economic Populism and Bandwagon Bigotry"; Haney-López, *Dog Whistle Politics*; Hochschild, *Strangers in Their Own Land*.
8. Strangleman, "Smokestack Nostalgia."
9. Rudacille, "How Toxic Is Smokestack Nostalgia?"; Strangleman, "Smokestack Nostalgia"; Berger, "Industrial Heritage."
10. Prno and Scott Slocombe, "Exploring the Origins of 'Social License to Operate.'"
11. Conde, "Resistance to Mining"; Temper et al., "Global Environmental Justice Atlas"; Muradian, Martinez-Alier, and Correa, "International Capital versus Local Population."
12. US Geological Survey, *Mineral Commodities Summaries 2016*.
13. Isidore, "Why U.S. Oil Production Is Booming"; Pulido et al., "Environmental Deregulation"; US Geological Survey, "Trump Administration Announces Strategy."
14. Kojola and Lequieu, "Performing Transparency, Embracing Regulations."
15. Gilberthorpe and Banks, "Development on Whose Terms?"; Mayes, McDonald, and Pini, "'Our' Community"; Humphreys, "Business Perspective"; Phadke, "Green Energy Futures"; Himley, "Mining History."
16. Phadke, "Green Energy Futures"; Mulvaney, *Solar Power Innovation*.
17. Hochschild, *Strangers in Their Own Land*; Ashwood, *For-Profit Democracy*.
18. Tsing, *Friction*.
19. Hjerpe, "Outdoor Recreation as a Sustainable Export Industry"; Stock and Bradt, "U.S. Forest Service Environmental Assessment."
20. Kojola, Xiao, and McCright, "Environmental Concern."
21. Montrie, "Expedient Environmentalism."
22. Barca, "On Working-Class Environmentalism"; Dreiling, "Remapping North American Environmentalism"; Gould, Lewis, and Roberts, "Blue-Green Coalitions."
23. Hanyes, *Dubious Alliance*.
24. However, the United Steelworkers went on to defend Reserve Mining when it was briefly shut down in the 1970s over the pollution. See Langston, *Sustaining Lake Superior*.
25. Burnes, "BlueGreen Alliance."
26. Stevis, Morena, and Krause, "Introduction."
27. United Steel Workers Canada, "Steelworkers Step Up Global Campaign."
28. Ramsay, "PolyMet Project Labor Agreement Signed."
29. Pearson et al., "Risks and Costs to Human Health."

BIBLIOGRAPHY

Abrams, Jesse, and John C. Bliss. "Amenity Landownership, Land Use Change, and the Re-creation of 'Working Landscapes.'" *Society & Natural Resources* 26, no. 7 (2013): 845–59. https://doi.org/10.1080/08941920.2012.719587.

Acharya, Ram N., Krishna P. Paudel, and L. Upton Hatch. "Impact of Nostalgia and Past Experience on Recreational Demand for Wilderness." *Applied Economics Letters* 16, no. 5 (2009): 449–53. https://doi.org/10.1080/13504850601032099.

Adam, Barbara. *Timescapes of Modernity: The Environment and Invisible Hazards*. London: Routledge, 1998.

Adams, Alison E., Thomas E. Shriver, Anne Saville, and Gary Webb. "Forty Years on the Fenceline: Community, Memory, and Chronic Contamination." *Environmental Sociology* 4, no. 2 (2018): 210–20. https://doi.org/10.1080/23251042.2017.1414660.

Adams, Zeno, and Thorsten Glück. "Financialization in Commodity Markets: A Passing Trend or the New Normal?" *Journal of Banking & Finance* 60 (2015): 93–111. https://doi.org/10.1016/j.jbankfin.2015.07.008.

Adelman, Bonnie Jane Eizen, Thomas A. Heberlein, and Thomas M. Bonnicksen. "Social Psychological Explanations for the Persistence of a Conflict between Paddling Canoeists and Motorcraft Users in the Boundary Waters Canoe Area." *Leisure Sciences* 5, no. 1 (1982): 45–61. https://doi.org/10.1080/01490408209512989.

Alario, Margarita, and William Freudenburg. "The Paradoxes of Modernity: Scientific Advances, Environmental Problems, and Risks to the Social Fabric?" *Sociological Forum* 18, no. 2 (2003): 193.

Albritton, Rachel, Taylor V. Stein, and Brijesh Thapa. "Exploring Conflict and Tolerance between and within Off-Highway Vehicle Recreationists." *Journal of Park & Recreation Administration* 27, no. 4 (2009).

Ali, Saleem. *Mining, the Environment, and Indigenous Development Conflicts*. Tucson: University of Arizona Press, 2003.

Allison, James Robert. *Sovereignty for Survival: American Energy Development and Indian Self-Determination*. New Haven, CT: Yale University Press, 2005.

Allister, Mark. Introduction to *Eco-Man: New Perspectives on Masculinity and Nature*, edited by Mark Allister, 1–13. Charlottesville: University of Virginia Press, 2004.

American Rivers. "America's Most Endangered Rivers 2015." 2015. www.americanrivers.org/.

Anderson, Carol. *White Rage: The Unspoken Truth of Our Racial Divide*. New York: Bloomsbury, 2016.

Anderson, Lewis Clarke. "The Copper-Nickel Controversy Or Can We Mine Without a Mess." *Minnesota Conservation Volunteer*, 1975.

Andrews, Eleanor, and James McCarthy. "Scale, Shale, and the State: Political Ecologies and Legal Geographies of Shale Gas Development in Pennsylvania." *Journal of Environmental Studies and Sciences* 4, no. 1 (2014): 7–16. https://doi.org/10.1007/s13412-013-0146-8.

Anshelm, Jonas, and Martin Hultman. "A Green Fatwā? Climate Change as a Threat to the Masculinity of Industrial Modernity." *NORMA* 9, no. 2 (2014): 84–96. https://doi.org/10.1080/18902138.2014.908627.

Anzalone Liszt Grove Research. "Minnesotans Strongly Oppose Sulfide Mining near the Boundary Waters Wilderness." Campaign to Save the Boundary Waters, March 8, 2016.

———. "Summary of Registered Voters in Minnesota." Campaign to Save the Boundary Waters, April 7, 2015.

Arbatli, Ekim. "Resource Nationalism Revisited: A New Conceptualization in Light of Changing Actors and Strategies in the Oil Industry." *Energy Research & Social Science* 40 (2018): 101–8. https://doi.org/10.1016/j.erss.2017.11.030.

Arboleda, Martín. "Financialization, Totality and Planetary Urbanization in the Chilean Andes." *Geoforum* 67 (2015): 4–13. https://doi.org/10.1016/j.geoforum.2015.09.016.

Arvin, Jariel. "The Indigenous-Led Fight to Stop the Line 3 Oil Pipeline Expansion in Minnesota, Explained." *Vox*, March 25, 2021. www.vox.com.

Ashwood, Loka. *For-Profit Democracy: Why the Government Is Losing the Trust of Rural America*. New Haven, CT: Yale University Press, 2018.

Backes, David. *Canoe Country: An Embattled Wilderness*. Minocqua: NorthWord, 1991.

Badiou, Allan, ed. *What Is a People*. New York: Columbia University Press, 2016.

Baeten, John, Nancy Langston, and Don Lafreniere. "A Spatial Evaluation of Historic Iron Mining Impacts on Current Impaired Waters in Lake Superior's Mesabi Range." *Ambio* 47, no. 2 (2018): 231–44. https://doi.org/10.1007/s13280-017-0948-0.

Baker, Lawrence A. "Potential Ecological Impacts of the Twin Metals Mine." Northeastern Minnesotans for Wilderness, November 24, 2013.

Baker, Zeke, Julia Ekstrom, and Louise Bedsworth. "Climate Information? Embedding Climate Futures within Temporalities of California Water Management." *Environmental Sociology* 4, no. 4 (2018): 419–33. https://doi.org/10.1080/23251042.2018.1455123.

Bakker, Karen, and Gavin Bridge. "Material Worlds? Resource Geographies and the 'matter of Nature.'" *Progress in Human Geography* 30, no. 1 (2006): 5–27. https://doi.org/10.1191/0309132506ph588oa.

Barca, Stefania. "On Working-Class Environmentalism: A Historical and Transnational Overview." *Interface* 4, no. 2 (2012): 61–80.

Barker, Adam J., and Jenny Pickerill. "Radicalizing Relationships to and through Shared Geographies: Why Anarchists Need to Understand Indigenous Connections to Land and Place." *Antipode* 44, no. 5 (2012): 1705–25. https://doi.org/10.1111/j.1467-8330.2012.01031.x.

Bartlett, Robert V. *The Reserve Mining Controversy: Science, Technology, and Environmental Quality*. Bloomington: Indiana University Press, 1980.
Barzen, Mimi. "Minnesota Forestry History Stories—Peak Logging Years." Minnesota Department of Natural Resources, 2011. www.dnr.state.mn.us.
Beamish, Thomas D. "Environmental Hazard and Institutional Betrayal: Lay-Public Perceptions of Risk in the San Luis Obispo County Oil Spill." *Organization & Environment*, 2016. https://doi.org/10.1177/1086026601141001.
Behsudi, Adam. "Minnesota on the Edge: 'I've Voted Democrat My Whole Life. It's Getting Tougher.'" *Politico*, March 22, 2020.
Bell, Michael Mayerfeld. *Childerley: Nature and Morality in a Country Village*. Chicago: University of Chicago Press, 1994.
Bell, Shannon Elizabeth. *Fighting King Coal: The Challenges to Micromobilization in Central Appalachia*. Cambridge, MA: MIT Press, 2016.
———. *Our Roots Run Deep as Ironweed: Appalachian Women and the Fight for Environmental Justice*. Urbana: University of Illinois Press, 2013.
Bell, Shannon Elizabeth, Jenrose Fitzgerald, and Richard York. "Protecting the Power to Pollute: Identity Co-Optation, Gender, and the Public Relations Strategies of Fossil Fuel Industries in the United States." *Environmental Sociology* 5, no. 3 (2019): 323–38. https://doi.org/10.1080/23251042.2019.1624001.
Bell, Shannon Elizabeth, and Richard York. "Community Economic Identity: The Coal Industry and Ideology Construction in West Virginia." *Rural Sociology* 75, no. 1 (2010): 111–43. https://doi.org/10.1111/j.1549-0831.2009.00004.x.
Benford, Robert D., and David A. Snow. "Framing Processes and Social Movements: An Overview and Assessment." *Annual Review of Sociology* 26, no. 1 (2000): 611–39. https://doi.org/10.1146/annurev.soc.26.1.611.
Bennett, W. Lance. *The Logic of Connective Action: Digital Media and the Personalization of Contentious Politics*. New York: Cambridge University Press, 2013.
Berger, Stefan. "Industrial Heritage and the Ambiguities of Nostalgia for an Industrial Past in the Ruhr Valley, Germany." *Labor: Studies in Working-Class Histories of the Americas* 16, no. 1 (2019): 37–64.
Berns, Gretchen Newhouse, and Steven Simpson. "Outdoor Recreation Participation and Environmental Concern: A Research Summary." *Journal of Experiential Education* 32, no. 1 (2009): 79–91. https://doi.org/10.1177/105382590903200107.
Besek, Jordan Fox. "On the Interactive Nature of Place-Making: Modifying Growth Machine Theory to Capture the Spatial and Temporal Connections That Spawned the Asian Carp Invasion." *The Sociological Quarterly*, no. 1 (2021): 121–42. https://doi.org/10.1080/00380253.2020.1715307.
Bierschbach, Briana. "How the Specter of the Decades-Long Fight over the BWCA Hangs over PolyMet." *MinnPost*, November 12, 2015. www.minpost.com.
Bingham, Clara, and Laura Leedy Gansler. *Class Action: The Landmark Case That Changed Sexual Harassment Law*. New York: Anchor Books, 2003.
Bjorhus, Jennifer. "Copper Mine Leases Denied: Feds Say Twin Metals Plan Poses Too Big a Risk to BWCA." *Star Tribune*, December 16, 2016.

———. "McCollum Fighting for Mine Study: Plug Pulled on Review after Trump Was Elected." *Star Tribune*, May 22, 2019.

———. "Mine Promises No Acid Drainage: Twin Metals Touts Its 'Dry Stack' Option; Opponents Say It Won't Protect BWCA." *Star Tribune*, July 19, 2019.

Bloomquist, Lee. "Company Still Hopes to Establish an Open-Pit Mine near Babbitt, Minn." *Duluth News-Tribune*, September 25, 2000.

Blunt, Alison. "Collective Memory and Productive Nostalgia: Anglo-Indian Home-making at McCluskieganj." *Environment and Planning D: Society and Space* 21, no. 6 (2003): 717–38. https://doi.org/10.1068/d327.

Bobo, Lawrence D. "Racism in Trump's America: Reflections on Culture, Sociology, and the 2016 US Presidential Election." *The British Journal of Sociology* 68 (2017): S85–104. https://doi.org/10.1111/1468-4446.12324.

Bonikowski, Bart. "Three Lessons of Contemporary Populism in Europe and the United States." *The Brown Journal of World Affairs* 23, no. 1 (2017): 9–24.

Bonikowski, Bart, and Noam Gidron. "The Populist Style in American Politics: Presidential Campaign Rhetoric, 1952–1996." *Social Forces* 94 (2016). https://doi.org/10.1093/sf/sov120.

Bonilla-Silva, Eduardo. *Racism without Racists: Color-Blind Racism and the Persistence of Racial Inequality in America*. 5th ed. Lanham, MD: Rowman and Littlefield, 2018.

Bonnett, Alastair. *Left in the Past: Radicalism and the Politics of Nostalgia*. New York: Continuum, 2010.

Bonnett, Alastair, and Catherine Alexander. "Mobile Nostalgias: Connecting Visions of the Urban Past, Present and Future amongst Ex-Residents." *Transactions of the Institute of British Geographers* 38, no. 3 (2013): 391–402. https://doi.org/10.1111/j.1475-5661.2012.00531.x.

Bosworth, Kai. "'They're Treating Us like Indians!': Political Ecologies of Property and Race in North American Pipeline Populism." *Antipode* 53, no. 3 (2021): 665–85. https://doi.org/10.1111/anti.12426.

Boucquey, Noëlle. "'That's My Livelihood, It's Your Fun': The Conflicting Moral Economies of Commercial and Recreational Fishing." *Journal of Rural Studies* 54 (2017): 138–50. https://doi.org/10.1016/j.jrurstud.2017.06.018.

Boudet, Hilary, Dylan Bugden, Chad Zanocco, and Edward Maibach. "The Effect of Industry Activities on Public Support for 'Fracking.'" *Environmental Politics* 25, no. 4 (2016): 593–612. https://doi.org/10.1080/09644016.2016.1153771.

Bourdieu, Pierre. *Reproduction in Education, Society and Culture*. 2nd ed. London: Sage, 1990.

———. "Social Space and Symbolic Power." *Sociological Theory* 7, no. 1 (1989): 14–25. https://doi.org/10.2307/202060.

Boym, Svetlana. *The Future of Nostalgia*. New York: Basic Books, 2001.

Braun, Carola. "Not in My Backyard: CCS Sites and Public Perception of CCS." *Risk Analysis* 37, no. 12 (2017): 2264–75. https://doi.org/10.1111/risa.12793.

Brecher, Jeremy, and the Labor Network for Sustainability. "Stormy Weather: Climate Change and a Divided Labor Movement." *New Labor Forum* 22, no. 1 (2013): 75–81. https://doi.org/10.1177/1095796012471308.

Brechin, Gray. "Conserving the Race: Natural Aristocracies, Eugenics, and the U.S. Conservation Movement." *Antipode* 28, no. 3 (1996): 229–45. https://doi.org/10.1111/j.1467-8330.1996.tb00461.x.

Bridge, Gavin. "Contested Terrain: Mining and the Environment." *Annual Review of Environment and Resources* 29, no. 1 (2004): 205–59. https://doi.org/10.1146/annurev.energy.28.011503.163434.

———. "Resource Geographies II: The Resource-State Nexus." *Progress in Human Geography* 38, no. 1 (2014): 118–30. https://doi.org/10.1177/0309132513493379.

Brininstool, Mark, and Daniel M. Flanagan. "2015 Minerals Yearbook: Copper." US Geological Society, October 2017.

Brodey, Sam. "Is Steel Dumping the Real Culprit for What Ails the Iron Range?" *MinnPost*, January 11, 2016. www.minnpost.com.

Bronfrenbrenner, Kate, and Tom Juravich. "The Evolution of Strategic and Coordinated Bargaining Campaigns in the 1990s: The Steelworkers Experience." In *Rekindling the Movement: Labor's Quest for Relevance in the 21st Century*, edited by Lowell Turner, Harry C. Katz, and Richard W. Hurd. Ithaca, NY: Cornell University Press, 2001.

Brooks, Jennifer. "Forest Service Scales Back Environmental Study of Mining near BWCA." *Star Tribune*. January 26, 2018.

Brown, Aaron. *Overburden: Modern Life on the Range*. Duluth, MN: Red Step, 2008.

Brubaker, Rogers. "Why Populism?" *Theory and Society* 46, no. 5 (2017): 357–85. https://doi.org/10.1007/s11186-017-9301-7.

Bullard, Robert D. *Dumping in Dixie: Race, Class, and Environmental Quality*. Boulder, CO: Westview, 1990.

———. "Ecological Inequities and the New South: Black Communities under Siege." *Journal of Ethnic Studies* 17 (1990): 101–15.

Bunker, Stephen G., and Paul S. Ciccantell. *Globalization and the Race for Resources*. Baltimore: Johns Hopkins University Press, 2005.

Burnes, Jerry. "DFL Considering Resolution 54." *Mesabi Daily News*, December 3, 2016.

———. "The BlueGreen Alliance: Working For The Iron Range?" *Mesabi Tribune*, February 21, 2017.

Burnham, Morey, Weston Eaton, Theresa Selfa, Clare Hinrichs, and Andrea Feldpausch-Parker. "The Politics of Imaginaries and Bioenergy Sub-Niches in the Emerging Northeast U.S. Bioenergy Economy." *Geoforum* 82 (2017): 66–76. https://doi.org/10.1016/j.geoforum.2017.03.022.

Burns, Shirley Stewart. *Bringing down the Mountains: The Impact of Mountaintop Removal Surface Coal Mining on Southern West Virginia Communities, 1970–2004*. Morgantown: West Virginia University Press, 2007.

Butler, Judith. "Reflections on Trump." *Fieldsights*, January 18, 2017. https://culanth.org.

Campaign to Save the Boundary Waters. "About the Campaign to Save the Boundary Waters." 2018. www.savetheboundarywaters.org.

———. "Timeline: Boundary Waters Canoe Wilderness and Campaign to Save the Boundary Waters." 2015.

Campbell, Gary, Laurajane Smith, and Margaret Wetherell. "Nostalgia and Heritage: Potentials, Mobilisations and Effects." *International Journal of Heritage Studies* 23, no. 7 (2017): 609–11. https://doi.org/10.1080/13527258.2017.1324558.

Carter, Bill. *Boom, Bust, Boom: A Story about Copper, the Metal That Runs the World.* New York: Scribner, 2012.

Caruso, Emily, Marcus Colchester, Fergus MacKay, Nick Hildyard, and Geoff Nettleton. *Extracting Promises: Indigenous Peoples, Extractive Industries and the World Bank.* Philippines: Tebtebba Foundation, 2003.

Casey, Edward S. *Getting Back into Place: Toward a Renewed Understanding of the Place-World.* Bloomington: Indiana University Press, 1993.

Center for Rural Policy and Development. *State of Rural Minnesota Report 2017.* Mankato, MN: Center for Rural Policy and Development, November 2016.

Center for Science in Public Participation. *The Potential for Acid Mine Drainage and Other Water Quality Problems at Modern Copper Mines Using State-of-the-Art Prevention, Treatment, and Mitigation Methods.* Bozeman, MT: Center for Science in Public Participation, November 20, 2014.

Chapin, Mac. "A Challenge to Conservationists." *World Watch Magazine*, 2004.

Chezick, Brent Timothy. "Let's Help the Anti-Mining Dems Lose." *Mesabi Daily News*, August 12, 2017.

Child, Brenda J. "The Absence of Indigenous Histories in Ken Burns's The National Parks: America's Best Idea." *The Public Historian* 33, no. 2 (2011): 24–29. https://doi.org/10.1525/tph.2011.33.2.24.

Clark, Brett. "The Indigenous Environmental Movement in the United States: Transcending Borders in Struggles against Mining, Manufacturing, and the Capitalist State." *Organization & Environment* 15, no. 4 (2002): 410–42. https://doi.org/10.1177/1086026602238170.

Clarke, Christopher E., Dylan Bugden, P. Sol Hart, Richard C. Stedman, Jeffrey B. Jacquet, Darrick T. N. Evensen, and Hilary S. Boudet. "How Geographic Distance and Political Ideology Interact to Influence Public Perception of Unconventional Oil/Natural Gas Development." *Energy Policy* 97 (2016): 301–9. https://doi.org/10.1016/j.enpol.2016.07.032.

Cole, Luke W, and Sheila R. Foster. *From the Ground Up: Environmental Racism and the Rise of the Environmental Justice Movement.* New York: New York University Press, 2001.

Coleman, John. "Iron Mining in Minnesota: A Difficult Time for Wild Rice." *A Chronicle of the Lake Superior Ojibwe, Mazina'igan*, 2018.

Collins, Patricia Hill. *Black Feminist Thought: Knowledge, Consciousness, and the Politics of Empowerment.* New York: Routledge, 1990.

———. "Toward a New Vision: Race, Class, and Gender as Categories of Analysis and Connection." *Race, Sex & Class* 1, no. 1 (1993): 25–45.

Conde, Marta. "Resistance to Mining: A Review." *Ecological Economics* 132 (2017): 80–90. https://doi.org/10.1016/j.ecolecon.2016.08.025.

Connell, Robert W. "A Whole New World: Remaking Masculinity in the Context of the Environmental Movement." *Gender and Society* 4, no. 4 (1990): 452–78.

Conservation Minnesota, Friends of the Boundary Waters Wilderness, Minnesota Center for Environmental Advocacy. "Frequently Asked Questions about Sulfide Mining in Minnesota: A Mining Truth Report." May 2012.

Coolican, J. Patrick. "Politicians Try to Bring Aid, Hope to the Iron Range." *Star Tribune*, December 21, 2015.

Coombe, Tom. "MINER Act Passes House." *Ely Echo*, December 1, 2017.

Cramer, Katherine J. *The Politics of Resentment: Rural Consciousness in Wisconsin and the Rise of Scott Walker*. Chicago: University of Chicago Press, 2016.

Crenshaw, Kimberlé Williams. "Demarginalizing the Intersection of Race and Sex: A Black Feminist Critique of Antidiscrimination Doctrine, Feminist Theory and Antiracist Politics." *University of Chicago Legal Forum*, 1989, 139–68.

———. "Mapping the Margins: Intersectionality, Identity Politics, and Violence against Women of Color." *Stanford Law Review* 43, no. 6 (1991): 1241–99. https://doi.org/10.2307/1229039.

Cronon, William. "The Trouble with Wilderness; or, Getting Back to the Wrong Nature." *Environmental History* 1, no. 1 (1996): 7–28. https://doi.org/10.2307/3985059.

———. *Uncommon Ground: Rethinking the Human Place in Nature*. New York: Norton, 1996.

Daggett, Cara. "Petro-Masculinity: Fossil Fuels and Authoritarian Desire." *Millennium* 47, no. 1 (2018): 25–44. https://doi.org/10.1177/0305829818775817.

Davidson, Debra J. "Emotion, Reflexivity and Social Change in the Era of Extreme Fossil Fuels." *The British Journal of Sociology* 70, no. 2 (2019): 442–62. https://doi.org/10.1111/1468-4446.12380.

Davies, Michael P. "Tailings Impoundment Failures: Are Geotechnical Engineers Listening?" *Waste Geotechnics*, 2002.

Davis, Fred. *Yearning for Yesterday: A Sociology of Nostalgia*. New York: Free Press, 1979.

Davis, Gerald F. *Managed by the Markets: How Finance Reshaped America*. Oxford: Oxford University Press, 2009.

Davis, Mike. "The Great God Trump and the White Working Class." *Catalyst* 1, no. 1 (2017). https://catalyst-journal.com.

Dear, Michael. "Understanding and Overcoming the NIMBY Syndrome." *Journal of the American Planning Association* 58, no. 3 (1992): 288–300. https://doi.org/10.1080/01944369208975808.

Deloria, Vine, and Clifford M. Lytle. *The Nations Within: The Past and Future of American Indian Sovereignty*. New York: Pantheon Books, 1984.

DeLuca, Kevin Michael, and Anne Demo. "Imagining Nature and Erasing Class and Race: Carleton Watkins, John Muir, and the Construction of Wilderness." *Environmental History* 6, no. 4 (2001): 541–60. https://doi.org/10.2307/3985254.

DePass, Dee. "New Trade Tariffs Thwart Steel Dumping, Help Iron Range." *Star Tribune*, September 14, 2016.

———. "Revival on the Range: Hope Unearthed." *Star Tribune*. November 6, 2006.

Desmond, Matthew. *On the Fireline: Living and Dying with Wildland Firefighters*. Chicago: University of Chicago Press, 2007.

Devine-Wright, Patrick. "Rethinking NIMBYism: The Role of Place Attachment and Place Identity in Explaining Place-Protective Action." *Journal of Community & Applied Social Psychology* 19, no. 6 (2009): 426–41. https://doi.org/10.1002/casp.1004.

Dewey, Scott. "Working for the Environment: Organized Labor and the Origins of Environmentalism in the United States, 1948–1970." *Environmental History* 3, no. 1 (1998): 45–63. https://doi.org/10.2307/3985426.

Dockstader, Sue, and Shannon Elizabeth Bell. "Ecomodern Masculinity, Energy Security, and Green Consumerism: The Rise of Biofuels in the United States:" *Critical Sociology* 46, nos. 4–5 (2019): 643–60. https://doi.org/10.1177/0896920519885010.

Doerfler, Jill, and Erik Redix. "Regional and Tribal Histories: The Great Lakes." In *The Oxford Handbook of American Indian History*, edited by Frederick E. Hoxie, 173–98. Oxford: Oxford University Press, 2016.

Dokshin, Fedor A. "Whose Backyard and What's at Issue? Spatial and Ideological Dynamics of Local Opposition to Fracking in New York State, 2010 to 2013." *American Sociological Review* 81, no. 5 (2016): 921–48. https://doi.org/10.1177/0003122416663929.

Dokshin, Fedor A., and Amanda Buday. "Not in Your Backyard! Organizational Structure, Partisanship, and the Mobilization of Nonbeneficiary Constituents against 'Fracking' in Illinois, 2013–2014." *Socius* 4 (2018): 1–17. https://doi.org/10.1177/2378023118783476.

Donges, Patrick, and Paula Nitschke. "Political Organizations and Their Online Communication." *Sociology Compass* 12, no. 2 (2017): 1–10. https://doi.org/10.1111/soc4.12554.

Dowie, Mark. *Conservation Refugees: The Hundred-Year Conflict between Global Conservation and Native Peoples*. Cambridge, MA: MIT Press, 2009.

Dreiling, Michael. "Remapping North American Environmentalism: Contending Visions and Divergent Practices in the Fight over NAFTA." *Capitalism, Nature, Socialism* 8, no. 4 (1997): 65–98. https://doi.org/10.1080/10455759709358766.

Drucker, Jeremy. "More than 200 Businesses Join Forces to Protect Minnesota's Boundary Waters Wilderness." Press release, Boundary Waters Business Coalition, Campaign to Save the Boundary Waters, February 13, 2017.

Dunbar, Elizabeth. "Alleged Risk to BWCA Roils PolyMet Mine Proposal." *MPR News*, September 2, 2015. www.mprnews.org.

Earl, Jennifer, Andrew Martin, John D. McCarthy, and Sarah A. Soule. "The Use of Newspaper Data in the Study of Collective Action." *Annual Review of Sociology* 30 (2004): 65–80. https://doi.org/10.1146/annurev.soc.30.012703.110603.

Earthworks. "Financial Assurance and Superfund: Who Should Pay for Mine Clean-Up, Industry or Taxpayers?" Accessed June 6, 2018. https://earthworks.org.

Eaton, Emily, and Abby Kinchy. "Quiet Voices in the Fracking Debate: Ambivalence, Nonmobilization, and Individual Action in Two Extractive Communities (Saskatchewan and Pennsylvania)." *Energy Research & Social Science* 20 (2016): 22–30. https://doi.org/10.1016/j.erss.2016.05.005.

Edsall, Thomas Byrne, and Mary D. Edsall. *Chain Reaction: The Impact of Race, Rights, and Taxes on American Politics*. New York: Norton, 1992.

Eleff, Robert M. "The 1916 Minnesota Miners' Strike against U.S. Steel." *Minnesota History*, Summer 1998, 63–74.

Eliasoph, Nina, and Paul Lichterman. "Culture in Interaction." *American Journal of Sociology* 108, no. 4 (2003): 735–94. https://doi.org/10.1086/367920.

Engels, Bettina, and Kristina Dietz. *Contested Extractivism, Society and the State: Struggles over Mining and Land*. London: Palgrave Macmillan, 2017.

Erlandson, Henry. "Why Is Minnesota's Democratic Party Called the DFL?" *Star Tribune*, January 25, 2020.

Escobar, Arturo. "Culture Sits in Places: Reflections on Globalism and Subaltern Strategies of Localization." *Political Geography* 20, no. 2 (2001): 139–74. https://doi.org/10.1016/S0962-6298(00)00064-0.

Estes, Nick. *Our History Is the Future: Standing Rock versus the Dakota Access Pipeline, and the Long Tradition of Indigenous Resistance*. New York: Verso, 2019.

Explore Minnesota. "Tourism and Minnesota's Economy." St. Paul, 2018.

Fahe. "Appalachian Poverty." Accessed June 12, 2016. www.fahe.org.

Farrell, Justin. *The Battle for Yellowstone: Morality and the Sacred Roots of Environmental Conflict*. Princeton, NJ: Princeton University Press, 2015.

———. *Billionaire Wilderness: The Ultra-Wealthy and the Remaking of the American West*. Princeton, NJ: Princeton University Press, 2020.

Feagin, Joe R. "Extractive Regions in Developed Countries: A Comparative Analysis of the Oil Capitals, Houston and Aberdeen." *Urban Affairs Review* 25, no. 4 (1990): 591–619. https://doi.org/10.1177/004208169002500405.

Fent, Ashley, and Erik Kojola. "Political Ecologies of Time and Temporality in Resource Extraction." *Journal of Political Ecology* 27, no. 1 (2020): 819–29. https://doi.org/10.2458/v27i1.23252.

Ferry, Elizabeth Emma, and Mandana E. Limbert. *Timely Assets: The Politics of Resources and Their Temporalities*. Santa Fe, NM: School for Advanced Research Press, 2008.

Filteau, Matthew R. "Who Are Those Guys? Constructing the Oilfield's New Dominant Masculinity." *Men and Masculinities* 17, no. 4 (2014): 396–416. https://doi.org/10.1177/1097184X14544905.

Finkel, Madelon L., and Jake Hays. "Environmental and Health Impacts of 'Fracking': Why Epidemiological Studies Are Necessary." *Journal of Epidemiology Community Health* 70, no. 3 (2016): 221–22. https://doi.org/10.1136/jech-2015-205487.

Finnegan, John R., and Jeffrey Mandel. "Final Report to the Legislature: Minnesota Taconite Workers Health Study." University of Minnesota School of Public Health, November 24, 2014.

Finney, Carolyn. *Black Faces, White Spaces: Reimagining the Relationship of African Americans to the Great Outdoors*. Chapel Hill: University of North Carolina Press, 2014.

Fond du Lac Band of Lake Superior Chippewa. "Complaint for Declaratory and Injunctive Relief Case No. 19-2489." September 10, 2019.

———. "Ojibwe Place Names." Onigamiinsing Dibaajimowinan—Duluth's Stories, 2016. www.duluthstories.net.

Fond du Lac Band of Lake Superior Chippewa, Grand Portage Band of Lake Superior Chippewa, Bois Forte Band of Chippewa, Great Lakes Indian Fish & Wildlife Commission, and the 1854 Treaty Authority. "How Will Cultural Resources Be Affected by the NorthMet Mine?" n.d.

Forgrave, Reid. "In Northern Minnesota, Two Economies Square Off: Mining vs. Wilderness." *New York Times*, October 12, 2017.

Foster, John Bellamy. "The Limits of Environmentalism without Class: Lessons from the Ancient Forest Struggle of the Pacific Northwest." *Capitalism, Nature, Socialism* 4 (1993): 11–40. https://doi.org/10.1080/10455759309358529.

Foucault, Michel. *The Archaeology of Knowledge and the Discourse on Language*. New York: Pantheon Books, 1972.

Frank, Thomas. *Listen, Liberal, or, What Ever Happened to the Party of the People?* New York: Picador, 2016.

Freedman, Eric. "When Indigenous Rights and Wilderness Collide: Prosecution of Native Americans for Using Motors in Minnesota's Boundary Waters Canoe Wilderness Area." *American Indian Quarterly* 26, no. 3 (2002): 378–92. https://doi.org/10.1353/aiq.2003.0037.

Freeman, Amy, and Dave Freeman. *A Year in the Wilderness: Bearing Witness in the Boundary Waters*. Minneapolis, MN: Milkweed, 2018.

Frelich, Lee E. "Forest and Terrestrial Ecosystem Impacts of Mining." Save the Boundary Waters, September 22, 2014.

Freudenburg, William R. "Addictive Economies: Extractive Industries and Vulnerable Localities in a Changing World Economy." *Rural Sociology* 57, no. 3 (1992): 305–32. https://doi.org/10.1111/j.1549-0831.1992.tb00467.x.

Freudenburg, William R., Scott Frickel, and Robert Gramling. "Beyond the Nature/Society Divide: Learning to Think about a Mountain." *Sociological Forum* 10, no. 3 (1995): 361–92. https://doi.org/10.1007/BF02095827.

Freudenburg, William R., and Robert Gramling. "Linked to What? Economic Linkages in an Extractive Economy." *Society & Natural Resources* 11, no. 6 (1998): 569–86. https://doi.org/10.1080/08941929809381103.

Frickel, Scott, and William R. Freudenburg. "Mining the Past: Historical Context and the Changing Implications of Natural Resource Extraction." *Social Problems* 43, no. 4 (1996): 444–66.

Friends of the Boundary Waters Wilderness. "How Cozy Is Twin Metals with the Trump Administration?" *Boundary Waters Blog*, March 5, 2019. www.friends-bwca.org.

Friends of the Boundary Waters Wilderness, Minnesota Center for Environmental Advocacy, Center for Biological Diversity, and Earth Justice. "Lawsuit Targets Minnesota's PolyMet Copper-Sulfide Mine Permit: Army Corps Authorized Largest Wetlands Destruction in State History." Press release, September 10, 2019.

Fruehan, Richard J., ed. *The Making, Shaping, and Treating of Steel*. 11th ed. Pittsburgh: AISE Steel Foundation, 1998.

FTSE Russell. "Company Report: Glencore PLC." Mergent Intellect, 2020.

Gaard, Greta Claire. *Ecofeminism: Women, Animals, Nature*. Philadelphia: Temple University Press, 1993.

Gamson, William A., and Andre Modigliani. "Media Discourse and Public Opinion on Nuclear Power: A Constructionist Approach." *American Journal of Sociology* 95, no. 1 (1989): 1–37. https://doi.org/10.1086/229213.

Gaventa, John. *Power and Powerlessness: Quiescence and Rebellion in an Appalachian Valley*. Urbana: University of Illinois Press, 1980.

Gedicks, Al. *The New Resource Wars: Native and Environmental Struggles against Multinational Corporations*. Boston: South End, 1993.

Gest, Justin, Tyler Reny, and Jeremy Mayer. "Roots of the Radical Right: Nostalgic Deprivation in the United States and Britain." *Comparative Political Studies* 51, no. 13 (2018): 1694–1719. https://doi.org/10.1177/0010414017720705.

Gestring, Bonnie. *U.S. Copper Porphyry Mines Report: The Track Record of Water Quality Impacts Resulting from Pipeline Spills, Tailings Failures, and Water Collection and Treatment Failures*. Washington, DC: Earthworks, 2012.

Ghose, Rina. "Big Sky or Big Sprawl? Rural Gentrification and the Changing Cultural Landscape of Missoula, Montana." *Urban Geography* 25, no. 6 (2004): 528–49. https://doi.org/10.2747/0272-3638.25.6.528.

Gieryn, Thomas F. "A Space for Place in Sociology." *Annual Review of Sociology* 26, no. 1 (2000): 463–96. https://doi.org/10.1146/annurev.soc.26.1.463.

Gilberthorpe, Emma, and Glenn Banks. "Development on Whose Terms? CSR Discourse and Social Realities in Papua New Guinea's Extractive Industries Sector." *Resources Policy* 37, no. 2 (2012): 185–93. https://doi.org/10.1016/j.resourpol.2011.09.005.

Gilchrist, Valerie J., and Robert L. Williams. "Key Informant Interviews." In *Doing Qualitative Research*, edited by Benjamin F. Crabtree and William L. Miller, 2nd ed., 71–88. Thousand Oaks, CA: Sage, 1999.

"Glencore, Steelworkers in Sudbury, Reach Deal." *Sudbury Star*, February 27, 2017. www.thesudburystar.com.

Goodstein, Eban S. *The Trade-Off Myth: Fact and Fiction about Jobs and the Environment*. Washington, DC: Island, 1999.

Goodwin, Jeff, and James M. Jasper, eds. *Rethinking Social Movements: Structure, Meaning, and Emotion*. Lanham, MD: Rowman and Littlefield, 2003.

Goodwin, Jeff, James M. Jasper, and Francesca Polletta. *Passionate Politics: Emotions and Social Movements*. Chicago: University of Chicago Press, 2001.

Gosnell, Hannah, and Jesse Abrams. "Amenity Migration: Diverse Conceptualizations of Drivers, Socioeconomic Dimensions, and Emerging Challenges." *GeoJournal* 76, no. 4 (2011): 303–22. https://doi.org/10.1007/s10708-009-9295-4.

Gottlieb, Robert. *Forcing the Spring: The Transformation of the American Environmental Movement*. Washington, DC: Island, 1993.

Gould, Kenneth A., Tammy L. Lewis, and Timmons J. Roberts. "Blue-Green Coalitions: Constraints and Possibilities in the Post 9-11 Political Environment." *Journal of World-Systems Research* 10, no. 1 (2004): 91–116. https://doi.org/10.5195/jwsr.2004.314.

Grattan, Laura. *Populism's Power: Radical Grassroots Democracy in America*. New York: Oxford University Press, 2016.

Gravelle, Timothy B., and Erick Lachapelle. "Politics, Proximity and the Pipeline: Mapping Public Attitudes toward Keystone XL." *Energy Policy* 83 (2015): 99–108. https://doi.org/10.1016/j.enpol.2015.04.004.

Green, Sarah, Chris Gregory, Madeleine Reeves, Jane K. Cowan, Olga Demetriou, Koch Insa, Carrithers Michael, et al. "Brexit Referendum: First Reactions from Anthropology." *Social Anthropology* 24, no. 4 (2016): 478–502.

Greer, Jed, and Kenny Bruno. *Greenwash: The Reality behind Corporate Environmentalism*. Lanham, MD: Rowman and Littlefield, 1998.

Grigsby, Mary. *Noodlers in Missouri: Fishing for Identity in a Rural Subculture*. Kirksville, MO: Truman State University Press, 2012.

Grossman, Zoltán. *Unlikely Alliances: Native Nations and White Communities Join to Defend Rural Lands*. Seattle: University of Washington Press, 2017.

Guarino, Ben. "Thousands of Montana Snow Geese Die after Landing in Toxic, Acidic Mine Pit." *Washington Post*, December 7, 2016.

Gusterson, Hugh. "From Brexit to Trump: Anthropology and the Rise of Nationalist Populism." *American Ethnologist* 44, no. 2 (2017): 209–14. https://doi.org/10.1111/amet.12469.

Guyer, Jane I. "Oil Assemblages and the Production of Confusion: Price Fluctuations in Two West African Oil-Producing Economies." In *Subterranean Estates: Life Worlds of Oil and Gas*, edited by Hannah Appel, Arthur Mason, and Michael Watts, 237–52. Ithaca, NY: Cornell University Press, 2015.

Hall, Stuart. "Authoritarian Populism: A Reply." *New Left Review* 1, no. 151 (1985): 115–24.

———. "Popular-Democratic vs Authoritarian Populism: Two Ways of 'Taking Democracy Seriously.'" In *Marxism and Democracy*, edited by Alan Hunt, 157–85. London: Lawrence and Wishart, 1980.

Hana, Bill. "PolyMet EIS Takes a Big Step." *Mesabi Daily News*, June 22, 2015.

Haney-López, Ian. *Dog Whistle Politics: How Coded Racial Appeals Have Reinvented Racism and Wrecked the Middle Class*. Oxford: Oxford University Press, 2014.

Hanyes, John Earl. *Dubious Alliance: The Making of Minnesota's DFL Party*. Minneapolis: University of Minnesota Press, 1984.

Haraway, Donna. *Simians, Cyborgs, and Women: The Reinvention of Nature*. New York: Routledge, 1991.

Harding, Sandra. *Whose Science? Whose Knowledge?* Ithaca, NY: Cornell University Press, 1991.

Harris, Cheryl I. "Whiteness as Property." *Harvard Law Review* 106, no. 8 (1993): 1707–91. https://doi.org/10.2307/1341787.

Hartsock, Nancy. *The Feminist Standpoint Revisited and Other Essays*. Boulder, CO: Westview, 1998.

Harvey, David. *A Brief History of Neoliberalism*. New York: Oxford University Press, 2005.

Helgeson, Baird. "Mine Project Tests DFL Unity." *Star Tribune*, December 15, 2013.

Helmberger, Marshall. "Court Hears Arguments for Supplemental Impact Statement." *Timberjay*, April 4, 2019.

———. "PolyMet Adds More Money to Cover Clean-Up of Mine Project." *Timberjay*, December 21, 2017.

———. "PolyMet's Financial Prospects Dim." *Timberjay*, March 28, 2018.

Hemphill, Stephanie. "Explaining the Iron Range Character." Minnesota Public Radio, September 19, 2005. http://news.minnesota.publicradio.org.

Himley, Matthew. "Mining History: Mobilizing the Past in Struggles over Mineral Extraction in Peru." *Geographical Review* 104, no. 2 (2014): 174–91. https://doi.org/10.1111/j.1931-0846.2014.12016.x.

Hjerpe, Evan E. "Outdoor Recreation as a Sustainable Export Industry: A Case Study of the Boundary Waters Wilderness." *Ecological Economics* 146 (2018): 60–68. https://doi.org/10.1016/j.ecolecon.2017.10.001.

Hobsbawm, Eric. "Introduction: Inventing Traditions." In *The Invention of Tradition*, edited by Eric Hobsbawm and Terence Ranger, 1–14. Cambridge: Cambridge University Press, 1983.

Hochschild, Arlie Russell. *Strangers in Their Own Land: Anger and Mourning on the American Right*. New York: New Press, 2016.

Hodgkin, Katherine, and Susannah Radstone, eds. *Contested Pasts: The Politics of Memory*. London: Routledge, 2003.

———. "Introduction: Contest Pasts." In *Contested Pasts: The Politics of Memory*, edited by Katherine Hodgkin and Susannah Radstone, 1–21. London: Routledge, 2003.

Holloway, Sarah L. "Burning Issues: Whiteness, Rurality and the Politics of Difference." *Geoforum* 38, no. 1 (2007): 7–20. https://doi.org/10.1016/j.geoforum.2006.01.004.

Holstein, James A., and Jaber F. Gubrium, eds. *Inside Interviewing: New Lenses, New Concerns*. Thousand Oaks, CA: Sage, 2003.

hooks, bell. *Ain't I a Woman: Black Women and Feminism*. Boston: South End, 1981.

Hoover, Elizabeth. *The River Is in Us: Fighting Toxics in a Mohawk Community*. Minneapolis: University of Minnesota Press, 2017.

Huber, Matthew T. *Lifeblood: Oil, Freedom, and the Forces of Capital*. Minneapolis: University of Minnesota Press, 2013.

Hultman, Martin. "The Making of an Environmental Hero: A History of Ecomodern Masculinity, Fuel Cells and Arnold Schwarzenegger." *Environmental Humanities* 2, no. 1 (2013): 79–99. https://doi.org/10.1215/22011919-3610360.

Humphreys, David. "A Business Perspective on Community Relations in Mining." *Resources Policy* 26, no. 3 (2000): 127–31. https://doi.org/10.1016/S0301-4207(00)00024-6.

Hurley, Patrick T., and Yılmaz Arı. "Mining (Dis)Amenity: The Political Ecology of Mining Opposition in the Kaz (Ida) Mountain Region of Western Turkey." *Development and Change* 42, no. 6 (2011): 1393–1415. https://doi.org/10.1111/j.1467-7660.2011.01737.x.

Inglehart, Ronald, and Pippa Norris. "Trump, Brexit, and the Rise of Populism: Economic Have-Nots and Cultural Backlash." Rochester, NY: Social Science Research Network, July 29, 2016.

Investing News Network. "10 Top Copper-Producing Companies," June 28, 2015. http://investingnews.com.

Inwood, Joshua F. J., and Anne Bonds. "Property and Whiteness: The Oregon Standoff and the Contradictions of the U.S. Settler State." *Space and Polity* 21, no. 3 (2017): 253–68. https://doi.org/10.1080/13562576.2017.1373425.

Iron Mining Association of Minnesota. "The Role of the IMA." Accessed May 10, 2021. www.taconite.org.

Isidore, Chris. "Why U.S. Oil Production Is Booming under Obama's Watch." CNN Business, January 28, 2015. https://money.cnn.com.

Jacob, Gerald R., and Richard Schreyer. "Conflict in Outdoor Recreation: A Theoretical Perspective." *Journal of Leisure Research* 12, no. 4 (1980): 368–80.

Jacobs, James A., Stephen M. Testa, and Jay H. Lehr. *Acid Mine Drainage, Rock Drainage, and Acid Sulfate Soils: Causes, Assessment, Prediction, Prevention, and Remediation*. Hoboken, NJ: Wiley Blackwell, 2014.

Jacobson, Ginger. "The Sociology of Emotions in a Contested Environmental Illness Case: How Gender and the Sense of Community Contribute to Conflict." *Environmental Sociology* 2, no. 3 (2016): 238–53. https://doi.org/10.1080/23251042.2016.1221169.

Jacoby, Karl. *Crimes against Nature: Squatters, Poachers, Thieves, and the Hidden History of American Conservation*. Berkeley: University of California Press, 2001.

Jasper, James M. *The Art of Moral Protest: Culture, Biography, and Creativity in Social Movements*. Chicago: University of Chicago Press, 1998.

Jerolmack, Colin, and Edward T. Walker. "Please in My Backyard: Quiet Mobilization in Support of Fracking in an Appalachian Community." *American Journal of Sociology* 124, no. 2 (2018): 479–516. https://doi.org/10.1086/698215.

Jobs for Minnesotans. "About Us." 2012. Accessed April 28, 2018. http://jobsforminnesotans.org.

Johnson, Cathryn, Timothy J. Dowd, and Cecilia L. Ridgeway. "Legitimacy as a Social Process." *Annual Review of Sociology* 32 (2006): 53–78. https://doi.org/10.1146/annurev.soc.32.061604.123101.

Jones, Owain, and Joanne Garde-Hansen, eds. *Geography and Memory: Explorations in Identity, Place and Becoming*. New York: Palgrave Macmillan, 2012.

Junod, Anne N., Jeffrey B. Jacquet, Felix Fernando, and Lynette Flage. "Life in the Goldilocks Zone: Perceptions of Place Disruption on the Periphery of the Bakken Shale." *Society & Natural Resources* 31, no. 2 (2018): 200–217. https://doi.org/10.1080/08941920.2017.1376138.

Kaunonen, Gary. *Flames of Discontent: The 1916 Minnesota Iron Ore Strike*. Minneapolis: University of Minnesota Press, 2017.

Kazis, Richard, Richard Lee Grossman, and Barry Commoner. *Fear at Work: Job Blackmail, Labor and the Environment*. Philadelphia: New Society, 1982.

Kelleher, Bob. "The Boundary Waters: 25 Years Later." Minnesota Public Radio, October 21, 2003.

Kennedy, Tony. "Looming End of Motorboats Lottery in BWCA Alarms Some Outfitters." *Star Tribune*, February 12, 2018.

Kess, David. *More than Just Ore: The Era That Really Made Ely*. Ely, MN: Ely-Winton Historical Society, 2014.

Kidd, Dustin, and Keith McIntosh. "Social Media and Social Movements." *Sociology Compass* 10, no. 9 (2016): 785–94. https://doi.org/10.1111/soc4.12399.

Kirsch, Stuart. *Mining Capitalism: The Relationship between Corporations and Their Critics*. Berkeley: University of California Press, 2014.

Kneas, David. "Subsoil Abundance and Surface Absence: A Junior Mining Company and Its Performance of Prognosis in Northwestern Ecuador." *Journal of the Royal Anthropological Institute* 22 (2016): 67–86. https://doi.org/10.1111/1467-9655.12394.

Kohl, Benjamin, and Linda Farthing. "Material Constraints to Popular Imaginaries: The Extractive Economy and Resource Nationalism in Bolivia." *Political Geography* 31, no. 4 (2012): 225–35. https://doi.org/10.1016/j.polgeo.2012.03.002.

Kojola, Erik. "Indigeneity, Gender and Class in Decision-Making about Risks from Resource Extraction." *Environmental Sociology* 5, no. 2 (2019): 130–48. https://doi.org/10.1080/23251042.2018.1426090.

———. "(Re)constructing the Pipeline: Workers, Environmentalists and Ideology in Media Coverage of the Keystone XL Pipeline." *Critical Sociology* 43, no. 6 (2017): 893–917. https://doi.org/10.1177/0896920515598564.

Kojola, Erik, and Amanda McMillan Lequieu. "Performing Transparency, Embracing Regulations: Corporate Framing to Mitigate Environmental Conflicts." *Environmental Sociology* 6, no. 4 (2020): 364–74. https://doi.org/10.1080/23251042.2020.1790717.

Kojola, Erik, Chenyang Xiao, and Aaron M. McCright. "Environmental Concern of Labor Union Members in the United States." *Sociological Quarterly* 55, no. 1 (2014): 72–91. https://doi.org/10.1111/tsq.12048.

Kraker, Dan. "Iron Range Voters Turn to Trump to Boost Region's Struggling Economy." *MPR News*, November 17, 2016. www.mprnews.org.

———. "Mine Layoffs Bring New Calls to Remake Iron Range Economy, but into What?" *MPR News*. April 11, 2016. www.mprnews.org.

Kreye, Melissa M., Elizabeth F. Pienaar, and Alison E. Adams. "The Role of Community Identity in Cattlemen Response to Florida Panther Recovery Efforts." *Society & Natural Resources* 30, no. 1 (2017): 79–94. https://doi.org/10.1080/08941920.2016.1180730.

Kubal, Timothy, and Rene Becerra. "Social Movements and Collective Memory." *Sociology Compass* 8, no. 6 (2014): 865–75. https://doi.org/10.1111/soc4.12166.

Kuipers, James R., Ann S. Maest, Kimberley A. MacHardy, and Gregory Lawson. *Comparison of Predicted and Actual Water Quality at Hardrock Mines: The Reliability of Predictions in Environmental Impact Statements*. Butte, MT: Kuipers and Associates; Buka Environmental, 2006.

Labban, Mazen. "Oil in Parallax: Scarcity, Markets, and the Financialization of Accumulation." In "Geographies of Peak Oil." Special issue. *Geoforum* 41, no. 4 (2010): 541–52. https://doi.org/10.1016/j.geoforum.2009.12.002.

Laclau, Ernesto. *On Populist Reason*. London: Verso, 2005.

Ladd, Anthony E. "Environmental Disputes and Opportunity-Threat Impacts Surrounding Natural Gas Fracking in Louisiana." *Social Currents* 1, no. 3 (2014): 293–311. https://doi.org/10.1177/2329496514540132.

Ladino, Jennifer K. "Longing for Wonderland: Nostalgia for Nature in Post-Frontier America." *Iowa Journal of Cultural Studies* 5, no. 1 (2004): 88–109. https://doi.org/10.17077/2168-569X.1118.

———. *Reclaiming Nostalgia: Longing for Nature in American Literature*. Charlottesville: University of Virginia Press, 2012.

LaDuke, Winona. *All Our Relations: Native Struggles for Land and Life*. Boston: South End, 1999.

LaDuke, Winona, and Brian Carlson. *Our Manoomin, Our Life: The Anishinaabeg Struggle to Protect Wild Rice*. Ponsford, MN: White Earth Land Recovery Project, 2003.

Lamont, Michèle, and Laurent Thévenot. *Rethinking Comparative Cultural Sociology: Repertoires of Evaluation in France and the United States*. Cambridge: Cambridge University Press, 2000.

Lamppa, Marvin G. *Minnesota's Iron Country: Rich Ore, Rich Lives*. Duluth, MN: Lake Superior Port Cities, 2004.

Landis, Paul H. *Three Iron Mining Towns: A Study in Cultural Change*. Middleton, WI: Social Ecology, 1997.

Langston, Nancy. *Sustaining Lake Superior: An Extraordinary Lake in a Changing World*. New Haven, CT: Yale University Press, 2017.

Lapakko, Kim A. "Prediction of Acid Mine Drainage from Duluth Complex Mining Wastes in Northeastern Minnesota." In *Proceedings of the 1988 Mine Drainage and Surface Mine Reclamation Conference*, 180–90. Pittsburgh: US Department of the Interior, Bureau of Mines, 1989.

Lapakko, Kim A., and David A. Antonson. *Duluth Complex Rock Dissolution and Mitigation Techniques: A Summary of 35 Years of DNR Research*. St. Paul: Minnesota Department of Natural Resources, February 2012.

Lapakko, Kim A., Michael C. Olson, and David A. Antonson. *Dissolution of Duluth Complex Rock from the Babbitt and Dunka Road Prospects: Eight-Year Laboratory Experiment*. St. Paul: Minnesota Department of Natural Resources, June 2013. http://files.dnr.state.mn.us.

Larsen, Soren C. "Place Identity in a Resource-Dependent Area of Northern British Columbia." *Annals of the Association of American Geographers* 94, no. 4 (2004): 944–60. https://doi.org/10.1111/j.1467-8306.2004.00442.x.

Larson, Eric C., and Richard S. Krannich. "'A Great Idea, Just Not near Me!' Understanding Public Attitudes about Renewable Energy Facilities." *Society & Natural Resources* 29, no. 12 (2016): 1436–51. https://doi.org/10.1080/08941920.2016.1150536.

LeCain, Timothy J. *Mass Destruction: The Men and Giant Mines That Wired America and Scarred the Planet*. New Brunswick, NJ: Rutgers University Press, 2009.

Lefebvre, Henri. *The Production of Space*. Oxford, UK: Blackwell, 1991.

Legg, Stephen. "Memory and Nostalgia." *Cultural Geographies* 11, no. 1 (2004): 99–107. https://doi.org/10.1191/1474474004eu296ed.

Lewin, Philip G. "'Coal Is Not Just a Job, It's a Way of Life': The Cultural Politics of Coal Production in Central Appalachia." *Social Problems* 66, no. 1 (2019): 51–68. https://doi.org/10.1093/socpro/spx030.

Lewis, Ronald. "Appalachian Restructuring in Historical Perspective: Coal, Culture and Social Change in West Virginia." *Urban Studies* 30, no. 2 (1993): 299–308. https://doi.org/10.1080/00420989320080301.

Li, Tania. *Land's End: Capitalist Relations on an Indigenous Frontier*. Durham, NC: Duke University Press, 2014.

Lipsitz, George. *The Possessive Investment in Whiteness: How White People Profit from Identity Politics*. Philadelphia: Temple University Press, 2018.

———. *Time Passages: Collective Memory and American Popular Culture*. Minneapolis: University of Minnesota Press, 1990.

Lipton, Eric, and Lisa Friedman. "Oil Was Central in Decision to Shrink Bears Ears Monument, Emails Show." *New York Times*, March 5, 2018.

Lobao, Linda, Minyu Zhou, Mark Partridge, and Michael Betz. "Poverty, Place, and Coal Employment across Appalachia and the United States in a New Economic Era." *Rural Sociology* 81, no. 3 (2016): 343–86. https://doi.org/10.1111/ruso.12098.

Loew, Patty, and James Thannum. "After the Storm: Ojibwe Treaty Rights Twenty-Five Years after the Voigt Decision." *American Indian Quarterly* 35, no. 2 (2011): 161–91. https://doi.org/10.5250/amerindiquar.35.2.0161.

Loomis, Erik. *Empire of Timber: Labor Unions and the Pacific Northwest Forests*. Cambridge: Cambridge University Press, 2015.

Lopez, Pia. "A Paddler's View: Time on Our Waters Reminds Us Why They Need to Be Protected." *Duluth News Tribune*, July 29, 2017.

Lovrien, Jimmy. "Minnesota's Only Solar Panel Manufacturer Seeks IRRR Loan to Boost Employment, Production." *Duluth News Tribune*, September 6, 2019.

Lowenthal, David. *The Past Is a Foreign Country*. Cambridge: Cambridge University Press, 1985.

MacGregor, Sherilyn. "A Stranger Silence Still: The Need for Feminist Social Research on Climate Change." *Sociological Review* 57, no. s2 (2009): 124–40. https://doi.org/10.1111/j.1467-954X.2010.01889.x.

Mah, Alice. *Industrial Ruination, Community, and Place: Landscapes and Legacies of Urban Decline*. Toronto: University of Toronto Press, 2012.

Malin, Stephanie A. *The Price of Nuclear Power: Uranium Communities and Environmental Justice*. New Brunswick, NJ: Rutgers University Press, 2015.

Malin, Stephanie A., and Kathryn Teigen DeMaster. "A Devil's Bargain: Rural Environmental Injustices and Hydraulic Fracturing on Pennsylvania's Farms." *Journal of Rural Studies* 47 (2016): 278–90. https://doi.org/10.1016/j.jrurstud.2015.12.015.

Malin, Stephanie A., Tara Opsal, Tara O'Connor Shelley, and Peter Mandel Hall. "The Right to Resist or a Case of Injustice? Meta-Power in the Oil and Gas Fields." *Social Forces* 97, no. 4 (2019): 1811–38. https://doi.org/10.1093/sf/soy094.

Manuel, Jeffrey T. "Efficiency, Economics, and Environmentalism: Low-Grade Iron Ore Mining in the Lake Superior District, 1913–2010." In *Mining North America: An Environmental History Since 1522*, edited by John R. McNeil and George Vrtis, 191–216. Oakland: University of California Press, 2017.

———. *Taconite Dreams: The Struggle to Sustain Mining on Minnesota's Iron Range, 1915–2000*. Minneapolis: University of Minnesota Press, 2015.

Marcotty, Josephine. "Agency Airs Concerns over Mine near BWCA." *Star Tribune*, June 14, 2016.

———. "Battle Waged over Mining Firms' Plans: A Debate over Mining, in Great Big Letters." *Star Tribune*, May 23, 2012.

———. "Before Copper Pit Opens, Expansion Debate Begins." *Star Tribune*, November 27, 2013.

———. "Cell Tower near BWCA Gets OK from Appeals Court." *Star Tribune*, June 18, 2012.

———. "Dayton Rebuffs Twin Metals Mine Proposal, Citing Risks to BWCA." *Star Tribune*, March 7, 2016.

———. "Lawsuit Alleges Lax Regulation of Major Minnesota Taconite Mine." *Star Tribune*, November 9, 2016.

———. "Mine Review Delayed Again." *Star Tribune*. August 24, 2013.

———. "Mine's Risks Spotlighted." *Star Tribune*. March 2, 2011.

———. "Minnesota's Mining Boom: New Riches or New Threat?" *Star Tribune*, September 25, 2011.

———. "PolyMet Clears a Hurdle with Minnesota Regulators, Though Battle Isn't Over." *Star Tribune*. November 10, 2015.

———. "PolyMet Copper Mine in Northeastern Minnesota Gets Cautious EPA Approval." *Star Tribune*, March 13, 2014.

Marley, Benjamin J. "The Coal Crisis in Appalachia: Agrarian Transformation, Commodity Frontiers and the Geographies of Capital." *Journal of Agrarian Change* 16, no. 2 (2016): 225–54. https://doi.org/10.1111/joac.12104.

Martinez-Alier, Joan. "The Environmentalism of the Poor." *Geoforum* 54 (2014): 239–41. https://doi.org/10.1016/j.geoforum.2013.04.019.

———. "Mining Conflicts, Environmental Justice, and Valuation." *Journal of Hazardous Materials, Risk and Governance* 86, nos. 1–3 (2001): 153–70. https://doi.org/10.1016/S0304-3894(01)00252-7.

Massey, Doreen. "A Global Sense of Place." In *Studying Culture*, edited by Ann Gray and Jim McGuigan, 232–340. London: Edward Arnold, 1997.

———. "Places and Their Pasts." *History Workshop Journal*, no. 39 (1995): 182–92. https://doi.org/10.1093/hwj/39.1.182.

———. *Space, Place, and Gender*. Minneapolis: University of Minnesota Press, 1994.

Mathews, Andrew S., and Jessica Barnes. "Prognosis: Visions of Environmental Futures." *Journal of the Royal Anthropological Institute* 22 (2016): 9–26. https://doi.org/10.1111/1467-9655.12391.

Matich, Teresa. "A Look at Historical Copper Prices." Investing News Network, April 13, 2016. http://investingnews.com.

Matthews, Todd L. "The Enduring Conflict of 'Jobs versus the Environment': Local Pollution Havens as an Integrative Empirical Measure of Economy Versus Environment." *Sociological Spectrum* 31, no. 1 (2010): 59–85. https://doi.org/10.1080/02732173.2011.525696.

Mayer, Adam. "Community Economic Identity and Colliding Treadmills in Oil and Gas Governance." *Journal of Environmental Studies and Sciences* 8 (8): 1–12. https://doi.org/10.1007/s13412-017-0435-8.

Mayes, Robyn, Paula McDonald, and Barbara Pini. "'Our' Community: Corporate Social Responsibility, Neoliberalisation, and Mining Industry Community Engagement in Rural Australia." *Environment and Planning A* 46, no. 2 (2014): 398–413. https://doi.org/10.1068/a45676.

McAdam, Doug, and Hilary Boudet. *Putting Social Movements in Their Place: Explaining Opposition to Energy Projects in the United States, 2000–2005*. Cambridge: Cambridge University Press, 2012.

McAdam, Doug, Hilary Schaffer Boudet, Jennifer Davis, Ryan J. Orr, W. Richard Scott, and Raymond E. Levitt. "'Site Fights': Explaining Opposition to Pipeline Projects in the Developing World." *Sociological Forum* 25, no. 3 (2010): 401–27. https://doi.org/10.1111/j.1573-7861.2010.01189.x.

McCarthy, James. "First World Political Ecology: Lessons from the Wise Use Movement." *Environment and Planning A* 34, no. 7 (2002): 1281–1302. https://doi.org/10.1068/a3526.

McGurty, Eileen. *Transforming Environmentalism: Warren County, PCBs, And the Origins of Environmental Justice*. New Brunswick, NJ: Rutgers University Press, 2007.

McHenry, Kristen Abatsis. "Getting Fracked: Gender Politics in Fracking Discourse." *Signs: Journal of Women in Culture and Society* 47, no. 1 (2021): 191–207. https://doi.org/10.1086/715229.

McQuarrie, Michael. "The Revolt of the Rust Belt: Place and Politics in the Age of Anger." *British Journal of Sociology* 68 (2017): S120–52. https://doi.org/10.1111/1468-4446.12328.

Meersman, Tom. "Proposed Copper-Nickel Mine Draws 'Extraordinary' Interest." *Star Tribune*, February 5, 2010.

Meier, Lars. "Metalworkers' Nostalgic Memories and Optimistic Official Representations of a Transformed Industrial Landscape." *The Sociological Review* 64, no. 4 (2016): 766–85. https://doi.org/10.1111/1467-954X.12391.

Melucci, Alberto. "The New Social Movements: A Theoretical Approach." *Social Science Information* 19, no. 2 (1980): 199–226. https://doi.org/10.1177/053901848001900201.

Merchant, Carolyn. *The Death of Nature: Women, Ecology, and the Scientific Revolution*. San Francisco: Harper and Row, 1980.

Messer, Chris M., Thomas E. Shriver, and Alison E. Adams. "Collective Identity and Memory: A Comparative Analysis of Community Response to Environmental Hazards." *Rural Sociology* 80, no. 3 (2015): 314–39. https://doi.org/10.1111/ruso.12069.

"Metals Mining Company Begins Minnesota's Permit-Seeking Process." *Duluth News-Tribune*, July 22, 2004.

Mills, Suzanne E. "Limitations to Inclusive Unions from the Perspectives of White and Aboriginal Women Forest Workers in the Northern Prairies." *Just Labour: A Canadian Journal of Work and Society* 11 (2007). https://doi.org/10.25071/1705-1436.88.

Minnesota Center for Environmental Advocacy. "Protecting Minnesota: Preventing a Disaster." *MCEA Newsletter*, 2015.

Minnesota Department of Employment and Economic Development. "Occupational Employment and Wage Statistics." Accessed July 24, 2022. https://mn.gov/deed.

———. "Quarterly Employment Demographics." Accessed August 8, 2022. https://mn.gov/deed.

Minnesota Department of Health. *Mesothelioma in Northeastern Minnesota and Two Occupational Cohorts: 2007 Update*. St. Paul: Center for Occupational Health and Safety, Chronic Disease and Environmental Epidemiology Section, December 7, 2007.

———. *Minnesota Climate and Health Profile Report 2015: An Assessment of Climate Change Impacts on the Health & Well-Being of Minnesotans*. St. Paul: Minnesota Department of Health, 2015.

———. "Minnesota Fish: Benefits and Risks." May 3, 2017. www.health.state.mn.us.

Minnesota Department of Natural Resources. *Inter-Agency Task Force Report on Base Metal Mining Impacts*. St. Paul: Minnesota Department of Natural Resources, January 1973.

———. "State Nonferrous Metallic Mineral Leasing Purposes and Policies." Accessed April 24, 2018. www.dnr.state.mn.us.

Minnesota Department of Natural Resources, US Army Corps of Engineers, and US Forest Service. "Factsheet: Tailings Basin Stability, NorthMet Mining Project and Land Exchange Final Environmental Impact Statement." St. Paul, 2015.

———. "Final Environmental Impact Statement (FEIS) NorthMet Mining Project and Land Exchange." St. Paul, November 2015.

———. "Final Environmental Impact Statement (FEIS) NorthMet Mining Project and Land Exchange—Appendix C: Tribal Agency Position Supporting Materials." St. Paul, November 2015.

———. "NorthMet Mining Project and Land Exchange Factsheet: Threatened and Endangered Species." St. Paul, 2015.

"Minnesota DNR Stops Work on Twin Metals Copper-Nickel Mine Project." *St. Paul Pioneer Press*, February 16, 2022.

Minnesota Environmental Quality Board. *The Minnesota Regional Copper-Nickel Study 1976–1979*. St. Paul: Minnesota Environmental Quality Board, August 31, 1979.

Minnesota Pollution Control Agency. "St. Louis River." Accessed April 30, 2018. www.pca.state.mn.us.

"Minnesota 2016 Presidential Caucus Results." *Star Tribune*, March 2, 2016. www.startribune.com.

Mische, Ann. "Measuring Futures in Action: Projective Grammars in the Rio + 20 Debates." *Theory and Society* 43, nos. 3–4 (2014): 437–64. https://doi.org/10.1007/s11186-014-9226-3.

Mishkind, Charles S. "Sexual Harassment Hostile Work Environment Class Actions: Is There Cause for Concern?" *Employee Relations Law Journal* 18, no. 1 (1992): 141–47.

Mitchell, Corey. "Minnesota Poll: Support Slipping for PolyMet Project." *Star Tribune*, September 20, 2014.

Mix, Tamara L., and Kristin G. Waldo. "Know(ing) Your Power: Risk Society, Astroturf Campaigns, and the Battle over the Red Rock Coal-Fired Plant." *Sociological Quarterly* 56, no. 1 (2014): 125–51. https://doi.org/10.1111/tsq.12065.

Moe, Richard. "Rushing to Ruin the Boundary Waters Wilderness." *New York Times*, May 17, 2018.

Moffitt, Benjamin. *The Global Rise of Populism: Performance, Political Style, and Representation*. Stanford, CA: Stanford University Press, 2016.

Mohai, Paul, David Pellow, and J. Timmons Roberts. "Environmental Justice." *Annual Review of Environment and Resources* 34, no. 1 (2009): 405–30. https://doi.org/10.1146/annurev-environ-082508-094348.

Molden, Berthold. "Resistant Pasts versus Mnemonic Hegemony: On the Power Relations of Collective Memory." *Memory Studies* 9, no. 2 (2016): 125–42. https://doi.org/10.1177/1750698015596014.

Montrie, Chad. "Expedient Environmentalism: Opposition to Coal Surface Mining in Appalachia and the United Mine Workers of America, 1945–1975." *Environmental History* 5, no. 1 (2000): 75–98. https://doi.org/10.2307/3985536.

———. *Making a Living: Work and Environment in the United States*. Chapel Hill: University of North Carolina Press, 2008.

Moore, Mik. "Coalition Building between Native American and Environmental Organizations in Opposition to Development: The Case of the New Los Padres Dam Project." *Organization & Environment* 11, no. 3 (1998): 287–313. https://doi.org/10.1177/0921810698113002.

Moreton-Robinson, Aileen. *The White Possessive: Property, Power, and Indigenous Sovereignty*. Minneapolis: University of Minnesota Press, 2015.

Morgan, Stephen L., and Jiwon Lee. "Economic Populism and Bandwagon Bigotry: Obama-to-Trump Voters and the Cross Pressures of the 2016 Election." *Socius* 5 (2019). https://doi.org/10.1177/2378023119871119.

———. "Trump Voters and the White Working Class." *Sociological Science* 5 (2018): 234–45. https://doi.org/10.15195/v5.a10.

Mouritsen, Karen E. "Decision: Leasing of Hardrock Minerals MNES 01352 and MNES 01353." US Bureau of Land Management, December 15, 2016.

Moyle, John B. "Some Chemical Factors Influencing the Distribution of Aquatic Plants in Minnesota." *American Midland Naturalist* 34, no. 2 (1945): 402–20.

Mudde, Cas. *Populist Radical Right Parties in Europe*. Cambridge: Cambridge University Press, 2007.

Muehlebach, Andrea. "The Body of Solidarity: Heritage, Memory, and Materiality in Post-Industrial Italy." *Comparative Studies in Society and History* 59, no. 1 (2017): 96–126. https://doi.org/10.1017/S0010417516000542.

Mui, Ylan Q. "Financial Turmoil Half a World Away Is Melting Minnesota's Iron Country." *Washington Post*, February 3, 2016.

Mukta, Parita, and David Hardiman. "The Political Ecology of Nostalgia." *Capitalism, Nature, Socialism* 11, no. 1 (2000): 113–33. https://doi.org/10.1080/10455750009358902.

Mulvaney, Dustin. *Solar Power Innovation, Sustainability, and Environmental Justice*. Berkeley: University of California Press, 2019.

Muradian, Roldan, Joan Martinez-Alier, and Humberto Correa. "International Capital versus Local Population: The Environmental Conflict of the Tambogrande Mining Project, Peru." *Society & Natural Resources* 16, no. 9 (2003): 775–92. https://doi.org/10.1080/08941920309166.

Myers, John. "Anti-Mining Rally Targets Duluth Chamber." *Duluth News-Tribune*, December 7, 2011.

———. "Critics' Poll Shows Growing Opposition to Copper Mining." *Duluth News-Tribune*, March 7, 2017.

———. "Dayton Calls Twin Metals Mine a Threat to the Boundary Water . . ." *Duluth News Tribune*, January 2, 2018.

———. "Emmer, Nolan Add Amendment to Defund Mining Study." *Duluth News Tribune*, September 7, 2017.

———. "Fed Shutdown Delays Review for PolyMet." *Duluth News-Tribune*. November 7, 2013.

———. "Keetac to Reopen: Workers to Return in January." *Duluth News Tribune*, December 29, 2016.

———. "PolyMet, Environmentalists Square Off over Proposed Copper Mine." *Duluth News-Tribune*, April 12, 2006.

———. "PolyMet Will Trade More Stock for Cash to Get Company through Permitting Stage." *Duluth News Tribune*, October 12, 2016.

———. "Twin Metals Gets Federal Mining Leases Back." *Duluth News-Tribune*, December 22, 2017.

Myers, Tom. *Technical Memorandum: Twin Metals Mining and the Boundary Waters Canoe Area Wilderness, Risk Assessment for Underground Metals Mining*. Ely: Northeastern Minnesotans for Wilderness, December 3, 2013.

Myrbo, Amy, Edward B. Swain, Dan R. Engstrom, Jill Coleman Wasik, James Brenner, Marta Dykhuizen Shore, Emily B. Peters, and G. Blaha. "Sulfide Generated by Sulfate Reduction Is a Primary Controller of the Occurrence of Wild Rice (Zizania Palustris) in Shallow Aquatic Ecosystems." *Journal of Geophysical Research: Biogeosciences* 122, no. 11 (2017): 2736–53. https://doi.org/10.1002/2017JG003787.

Nash, Steve. *Grand Canyon for Sale: Public Lands versus Private Interests in the Era of Climate Change*. Oakland: University of California Press, 2017.

Natural Resources Research Institute. "NRRI Geologists Define Minnesota Resources for Critical Minerals." *NRRI Now*, 2008.

Nelson, Peter B. "Rural Restructuring in the American West: Land Use, Family and Class Discourses." *Journal of Rural Studies* 17, no. 4 (2001): 395–407. https://doi.org/10.1016/S0743-0167(01)00002-X.

Nemanic, Mary Lou. *One Day for Democracy: Independence Day and the Americanization of Iron Range Immigrants*. Athens: Ohio University Press, 2007.

Nesper, Larry. *The Walleye War: The Struggle for Ojibwe Spearfishing and Treaty Rights*. Lincoln: University of Nebraska Press, 2002.

Neumann, Pamela. "Toxic Talk and Collective (In)Action in a Company Town: The Case of La Oroya, Peru." *Social Problems* 63, no. 3 (2016): 431–46. https://doi.org/10.1093/socpro/spw010.

Niemonen, Jack. "The Emotional Politics of Racism: How Feelings Trump Facts in an Era of Colorblindness." *Contemporary Sociology* 46, no. 1 (2017): 87–89. https://doi.org/10.1177/0094306116681813hh.

"No Extra Mine Comment Time." *Star Tribune*, February 28, 2014.

Nolan, Rick. "Nolan Brings Down the Hammer on Illegal Foreign Steel." Press release, August 25, 2016. https://nolan.house.gov.

Norgaard, Kari Marie. "Climate Denial and the Construction of Innocence: Reproducing Transnational Environmental Privilege in the Face of Climate Change." *Race, Gender & Class* 19, nos. 1–2 (2012): 80–103.

———. *Living in Denial: Climate Change, Emotions, and Everyday Life*. Cambridge, MA: MIT Press, 2011.

———. "'People Want to Protect Themselves a Little Bit': Emotions, Denial, and Social Movement Nonparticipation." *Sociological Inquiry* 76, no. 3 (2006): 372–96. https://doi.org/10.1111/j.1475-682X.2006.00160.x.

———. *Salmon and Acorns Feed Our People: Colonialism, Nature, and Social Action*. New Brunswick, NJ: Rutgers University Press, 2019.

Norgaard, Kari Marie, and Ron Reed. "Emotional Impacts of Environmental Decline: What Can Native Cosmologies Teach Sociology about Emotions and

Environmental Justice?" *Theory and Society* 46 (2017): 463–95. https://doi.org/10.1007/s11186-017-9302-6.
Norrgard, Chantal. *Seasons of Change: Labor, Treaty Rights, and Ojibwe Nationhood.* Chapel Hill: University of North Carolina Press, 2014.
"Now What?" Editorial. *Ely Echo*, June 30, 2017.
Oakes, Larry. "North Country Blues: Eveleth and Other Mining Towns in Northeastern Minnesota Have Seen Their Populations Age and Shrink." *Star Tribune*, May 20, 2001.
Ode, Kim. "Testing Their Boundary." *Star Tribune*, September 19, 2017.
Office of Minnesota Secretary of State. "2016 General Election Results." Accessed April 24, 2018. www.sos.state.mn.us.
Olick, Jeffrey K. "'Collective Memory': A Memoir and Prospect." *Memory Studies* 1, no. 1 (2008): 23–29. https://doi.org/10.1177/1750698007083885.
———. *The Collective Memory Reader*. New York: Oxford University Press, 2011.
Olick, Jeffrey K., and Joyce Robbins. "Social Memory Studies: From 'Collective Memory' to the Historical Sociology of Mnemonic Practices." *Annual Review of Sociology* 24, no. 1 (1998): 105–40. https://doi.org/10.1146/annurev.soc.24.1.105.
Oliver, Eric J., and Wendy M. Rahn. "Rise of the Trumpenvolk: Populism in the 2016 Election." *Annals of the American Academy of Political and Social Science* 667, no. 1 (2016): 189–206. https://doi.org/10.1177/0002716216662639.
Onello, Emily, Deb Allert, Steve Bauer, John Ipsen, Margaret Saracino, Kris Wegerson, Douglas Wendland, and Jennifer Pearson. "Sulfide Mining and Human Health in Minnesota." *Minnesota Medicine*, November–December 2016, 51–55.
Orenstein, Walker. "PolyMet Is Now Owned by Switzerland's Glencore. Why It Matters." *MinnPost*, June 28, 2019. www.minnpost.com.
Paap, Kris. "How Good Men of the Union Justify Inequality: Dilemmas of Race and Labor in the Building Trades." *Labor Studies Journal* 33, no. 4 (2008): 371–92. https://doi.org/10.1177/0160449X08322773.
Packer, George. "Hillary Clinton and the Populist Revolt." *New Yorker*, October 24, 2016.
Pantland, Walton. "Glencore: The Commodities Giant with No Soul." IndustriALL Global Union, April 25, 2018.
Parshley, Lois. "9 Places to Go to Enjoy the Great Outdoors." *National Geographic Adventure*, September 26, 2016. www.nationalgeographic.com.
Pasternak, Shiri. *Grounded Authority: The Algonquins of Barriere Lake against the State.* Minneapolis: University of Minnesota Press, 2017.
Pearson, Jennifer, John Ipsen, Steven Sutherland, Kristan Wegerson, and Emily Onello. "Risks and Costs to Human Health of Sulfide-Ore Mining near the Boundary Waters Canoe Area Wilderness." *Human and Ecological Risk Assessment: An International Journal* 26, no. 5 (2020): 1329–40. https://doi.org/10.1080/10807039.2019.1576026.
Peck, Jamie, and Henry Wai-Chung Yeung. *Remaking the Global Economy: Economic-Geographical Perspectives*. London: Sage, 2003.

Pellow, David N. *What Is Critical Environmental Justice?* Cambridge, UK: Polity, 2017.

Pellow, David N., and Lisa Sun-Hee Park. *The Silicon Valley of Dreams: Environmental Injustice, Immigrant Workers, and the High-Tech Global Economy*. New York: New York University Press, 2002.

Phadke, Roopali. "Green Energy Futures: Responsible Mining on Minnesota's Iron Range." *Energy Research & Social Science* 35 (2018): 163–73. https://doi.org/10.1016/j.erss.2017.10.036.

———. "Resisting and Reconciling Big Wind: Middle Landscape Politics in the New American West." *Antipode* 43, no. 3 (June 1, 2011): 754–76. https://doi.org/10.1111/j.1467-8330.2011.00881.x.

Pickering, Michael, and Emily Keightley. "The Modalities of Nostalgia." *Current Sociology* 54, no. 6 (2006): 919–41. https://doi.org/10.1177/0011392106068458.

Pijpers, Robert Jan, and Thomas Hylland Eriksen, eds. *Mining Encounters: Extractive Industries in an Overheated World*. London: Pluto, 2019.

Pliml, George. "Despite Concerns, Staying Blue." *Mesabi Daily News*, August 19, 2017.

Plumwood, Val. *Feminism and the Mastery of Nature*. London: Routledge, 1993.

Polletta, Francesca, and James M. Jasper. "Collective Identity and Social Movements." *Annual Review of Sociology* 27, no. 1 (2001): 283–305. https://doi.org/10.1146/annurev.soc.27.1.283.

PolyMet. "Community and Economic Benefits." 2016. Accessed May 10, 2021. https://polymetmining.com.

Prescod, Paul. "We Can't Abandon the Building Trades Unions to the Right." *Jacobin*, March 3, 2020.

Prno, Jason, and D. Scott Slocombe. "Exploring the Origins of 'Social License to Operate' in the Mining Sector: Perspectives from Governance and Sustainability Theories." *Resources Policy* 37, no. 3 (2012): 346–57. https://doi.org/10.1016/j.resourpol.2012.04.002.

Proescholdt, Kevin, Rip Rapson, and Miron L. Heinselman. *Troubled Waters: The Fight for the Boundary Waters Canoe Area Wilderness*. St. Cloud, MN: North Star, 1995.

Prudham, Scott W. *Knock on Wood: Nature as Commodity in Douglas-Fir Country*. New York: Routledge, 2005.

Pulido, Laura, Tianna Bruno, Cristina Faiver-Serna, and Cassandra Galentine. "Environmental Deregulation, Spectacular Racism, and White Nationalism in the Trump Era." *Annals of the American Association of Geographers* 109, no. 2 (2019): 520–32. https://doi.org/10.1080/24694452.2018.1549473.

Ramirez, Emil. "Both Sides Agree: Protect Environment—Good Jobs, Pristine Nature Can Coexist." *Duluth News Tribune*, February 16, 2018.

Ramsay, Charles. "PolyMet Project Labor Agreement Signed." *Mesabi Tribune*, August 24, 2007.

Ramstad, Evan. "PolyMet Receives $14 Million in Capital from Glencore." *Star Tribune*, June 16, 2016.

Ranco, Darren, and Dean Suagee. "Tribal Sovereignty and the Problem of Difference in Environmental Regulation: Observations on 'Measured Separatism' in Indian

Country." *Antipode* 39, no. 4 (2007): 691–707. https://doi.org/10.1111/j.1467-8330.2007.00547.x.

Raster, Amanda, and Christina Gish Hill. "The Dispute over Wild Rice: An Investigation of Treaty Agreements and Ojibwe Food Sovereignty." *Agriculture and Human Values* 34, no. 2 (2017): 267–81. https://doi.org/10.1007/s10460-016-9703-6.

Raynes, Dakota K. T., Tamara L. Mix, Angela Spotts, and Ariel Ross. "An Emotional Landscape of Place-Based Activism: Exploring the Dynamics of Place and Emotion in Antifracking Actions." *Humanity & Society* 40, no. 4 (2016): 401–23. https://doi.org/10.1177/0160597616669757.

Rebuffoni, Dean. "Kennecott to Take Over Stalled Copper Project." *Star Tribune*, May 26, 1982.

Rivera, Pia. "Copper Is Up on a Six-Month High." *Investing News*, November 7, 2016. http://investingnews.com.

Robbins, Paul, Katharine Meehan, Hannah Gosnell, and Susan J. Gilbertz. "Writing the New West: A Critical Review." *Rural Sociology* 74, no. 3 (2009): 356–82. https://doi.org/10.1526/003601109789037240.

Roberts, Ian. "Collective Representations, Divided Memory and Patterns of Paradox: Mining and Shipbuilding." *Sociological Research Online* 12, no. 6 (2008): 1–19. https://doi.org/10.5153/sro.1611.

Roediger, David R. *The Wages of Whiteness: Race and the Making of the American Working Class*. London: Verso, 1991.

———. "What If Labor Were Not White and Male? Recentering Working-Class History and Reconstructing Debate on the Unions and Race." *International Labor and Working-Class History* 51 (1997): 72–95. https://doi.org/10.1017/S014754790000199X.

Rolston, Jessica Smith. *Mining Coal and Undermining Gender: Rhythms of Work and Family in the American West*. New Brunswick, NJ: Rutgers University Press, 2014.

Rootes, Christopher. "Acting Locally: The Character, Contexts and Significance of Local Environmental Mobilisations." *Environmental Politics* 16, no. 5 (2007): 722–41. https://doi.org/10.1080/09644010701640460.

Rose, Fred. *Coalitions across the Class Divide: Lessons from the Labor, Peace, and Environmental Movements*. Ithaca, NY: Cornell University Press, 2000.

Ross, Gavin. "Copper, Nickel, Lead & Zinc Mining in the US." Industry report. IBISWorld, March 2020.

Ross, Jenna. "Another Small-Town Minnesota Grocery Store Calls It Quits: Aurora Residents Are Saying So Long to Zup's as Rural Shopping Habits Shift." *Star Tribune*, January 11, 2016.

Rossman, Gretchen B., and Sharon F. Rallis. *An Introduction to Qualitative Research: Learning in the Field*. Thousand Oaks, CA: Sage, 2017.

Rowell, Andrew. *Green Backlash: Global Subversion of the Environmental Movement*. London: Routledge, 1996.

Rudacille, Deborah. "How Toxic Is Smokestack Nostalgia?" *Aeon*, April 23, 2015. https://aeon.co.

Sassen, Saskia. *Globalization and Its Discontents: Essays on the New Mobility of People and Money*. New York: New Press, 1998.
Satterfield, Terre. *Anatomy of a Conflict: Identity, Knowledge, and Emotion in Old-Growth Forests*. Vancouver: University of British Columbia Press, 2002.
Sayer, Andrew. "Moral Economy and Political Economy." *Studies in Political Economy* 61 (2000): 79–103. https://doi.org/10.1080/19187033.2000.11675254.
Schaffartzik, Anke, Andreas Mayer, Nina Eisenmenger, and Fridolin Krausmann. "Global Patterns of Metal Extractivism, 1950–2010: Providing the Bones for the Industrial Society's Skeleton." *Ecological Economics* 122 (2016): 101–10. https://doi.org/10.1016/j.ecolecon.2015.12.007.
Scheman, Naomi. *Shifting Ground: Knowledge and Reality, Transgression and Trustworthiness*. New York: Oxford University Press, 2011.
Scheyder, Ernest, and Barbara Lewis. "Glencore's Risk Appetite Dwindles, Fueling Focus on Safer Regions." *Reuters*, September 5, 2019. https://www.reuters.com.
Schnaiberg, Allan, and Kenneth Alan Gould. *Environment and Society: The Enduring Conflict*. New York: St. Martin's, 1994.
Schuldt, Nancy, Jennifer Ballinger, Nikki Crowe, Wayne Dupuis, Kelly Emmons, Crystall Greensky, Emily Onello, Kristin Raab, and Melissa Walls. "Expanding the Narrative of Tribal Health: The Effects of Wild Rice Water Quality Rule Changes on Tribal Health Fond Du Lac Band of Lake Superior Chippewa Health Impact Assessment." Fond du Lac Band of Lake Superior Chippewa, 2018.
Scoones, Ian, Marc Edelman, Saturnino M. Borras Jr., Ruth Hall, Wendy Wolford, and Ben White. "Emancipatory Rural Politics: Confronting Authoritarian Populism." *The Journal of Peasant Studies* 45, no. 1 (2018): 1–20. https://doi.org/10.1080/03066150.2017.1339693.
Scott, Rebecca R. "Dependent Masculinity and Political Culture in Pro-Mountaintop Removal Discourse; or, How I Learned to Stop Worrying and Love the Dragline." *Feminist Studies* 33, no. 3 (2007): 484–509. https://doi.org/10.2307/20459158.
———. "Environmental Affects: NASCAR, Place and White American Cultural Citizenship." *Social Identities* 19, no. 1 (2013): 13–31. https://doi.org/10.1080/13504630.2012.753342.
———. *Removing Mountains: Extracting Nature and Identity in the Appalachian Coalfields*. Minneapolis: University of Minnesota Press, 2010.
———. "The Sociology of Coal Hollow: Safety, Othering, and Representations of Inequality." *Journal of Appalachian Studies* 15, nos. 1–2 (2009): 7–25. www.jstor.org/stable/41446816.
Searle, Newell R. *Saving Quetico-Superior: A Land Set Apart*. St. Paul: Minnesota Historical Society, 1977.
Sewell, William H., Jr. "A Theory of Structure: Duality, Agency, and Transformation." *American Journal of Sociology* 98, no. 1 (1992): 1–29. https://doi.org/10.1086/229967.
Shaffer, David. "PolyMet Committed to Disputed Mine Plan." *Star Tribune*, June 26, 2010.

———. "PolyMet Mining Hires Former MPCA Commissioner Moore." *Star Tribune*, January 26, 2011.
———. "Range Copper Firms atop 'Mega-Deposit' to Merge." *Star Tribune*, December 21, 2010.
Sheridan, Thomas E. "Embattled Ranchers, Endangered Species, and Urban Sprawl: The Political Ecology of the New American West." *Annual Review of Anthropology* 36, no. 1 (2007): 121–38. https://doi.org/10.1146/annurev.anthro.36.081406.094413.
Sherman, Jennifer. "Coping with Rural Poverty: Economic Survival and Moral Capital in Rural America." *Social Forces* 85, no. 2 (2006): 891–913. https://doi.org/10.1353/sof.2007.0026.
———. *Dividing Paradise: Rural Inequality and the Diminishing American Dream*. Berkeley: University of California Press, 2021.
Sherry, Allison. "The Eighth Congressional District." *Star Tribune*, June 8, 2014.
———. "Rick Nolan Wins Again over Stewart Mills in Tight, Expensive Minn. Eighth District Race." *Star Tribune*. November 9, 2016.
Shriver, Thomas E., Alison E. Adams, and Sherry Cable. "Discursive Obstruction and Elite Opposition to Environmental Activism in the Czech Republic." *Social Forces* 91, no. 3 (2013): 873–93. https://doi.org/10.1093/sf/sos183.
Shumway, J. Matthew, and Richard H. Jackson. "Place Making, Hazardous Waste, and the Development of Tooele County, Utah." *Geographical Review* 98, no. 4 (2008): 433–55. https://doi.org/10.1111/j.1931-0846.2008.tb00311.x.
Simoes, Alexander. "Copper Ore." Observatory of Economic Complexity, 2017. https://atlas.media.mit.edu.
———. "Nickel Ore." Observatory of Economic Complexity, 2017. https://atlas.media.mit.edu.
Simons, Abby. "Mining Face-Off." *Star Tribune*, August 24, 2014.
Simpson, Audra. *Mohawk Interruptus: Political Life across the Borders of Settler States*. Durham, NC: Duke University Press, 2014.
Simpson, Leanne Betasamosake. *As We Have Always Done: Indigenous Freedom through Radical Resistance*. Minneapolis: University of Minnesota Press, 2017.
Skocpol, Theda. *The Tea Party and the Remaking of Republican Conservatism*. New York: Oxford University Press, 2012.
Smith, Anthony D. *National Identity*. Reno: University of Nevada Press, 1991.
Smith, Laurajane, and Gary Campbell. "'Nostalgia for the Future': Memory, Nostalgia and the Politics of Class." *International Journal of Heritage Studies* 23, no. 7 (2017): 612–27. https://doi.org/10.1080/13527258.2017.1321034.
Snow, David A., E. Burke Rochford Jr., Steven K. Worden, and Robert D. Benford. "Frame Alignment Processes, Micromobilization, and Movement Participation." *American Sociological Review* 51, no. 4 (1986): 464–81. https://doi.org/10.2307/2095581.
Soja, Edward. *Postmodern Geographies: The Reassertion of Space in Critical Social Theory*. London: Verso, 1989.

Spence, Mark David. *Dispossessing the Wilderness: Indian Removal and the Making of the National Parks*. Oxford: Oxford University Press, 1999.

Spice, Anne. "Fighting Invasive Infrastructures: Indigenous Relations against Pipelines." *Environment and Society* 9, no. 1 (2018): 40–56. https://doi.org/10.3167/ares.2018.090104.

St. Anthony, Neal. "Officials Tout Benefits of Mine near Ely." *Star Tribune*, August 4, 2010.

Stark, Heidi Kiiwetinepinesiik. "Marked by Fire: Anishinaabe Articulations of Nationhood in Treaty Making with the United States and Canada." *American Indian Quarterly* 36, no. 2 (2012): 119–49. https://doi.org/muse.jhu.edu/article/470228.

———. "Respect, Responsibility, and Renewal: The Foundations of Anishinaabe Treaty Making with the United States and Canada." *American Indian Culture and Research Journal* 34, no. 2 (2010): 145–64. https://doi.org/10.17953/aicr.34.2.j0414503108l8771.

Steine, Cynthia. "Thoughts on Mining's Past, Its Future Potential on the Range." *Home Town Focus*, February 23, 2018. www.hometownfocus.us.

Stevis, Dimitris. "Deep Cleavages amongst US Labour Unions with Respect to Climate Change, Finds Report." Adapting Canadian Work and Workplaces, York University, Toronto, 2019. www.adaptingcanadianwork.ca.

Stevis, Dimitris, Edouard Morena, and Dunja Krause. "Introduction: The Genealogy and Contemporary Politics of Just Transitions." In *Just Transitions*, edited by Dimitris Stevis, Edouard Morena, and Dunja Krause, 1–31. London: Pluto, 2020.

St. George, Louie. "A Long-Range Issue: As the Iron Range Job Market Has Waned, So Have School Enrollments and Victories." *Duluth News-Tribune*, August 20, 2016.

Stock, James H., and Jacob T. Bradt. "U.S. Forest Service (USFS) Environmental Assessment (EA) on Proposed 20-Year Mineral Leasing Withdrawal in Superior National Forest." Harvard University, Cambridge, MA, August 8, 2018.

Stone, Andrew B. "Treaty of La Pointe, 1854." *MNopedia* (Minnesota Historical Society), September 30, 2014. www.mnopedia.org.

Strangleman, Tim. "'Smokestack Nostalgia,' 'Ruin Porn' or Working-Class Obituary: The Role and Meaning of Deindustrial Representation." *International Labor and Working-Class History* 84 (2013): 23–37. https://doi.org/10.1017/S0147547913000239.

Sturgeon, Noël. *Ecofeminist Natures: Race, Gender, Feminist Theory, and Political Action*. New York: Routledge, 1997.

Sweeney, Sean. "Contested Futures: Labor after Keystone XL." *New Labor Forum* 25, no. 2 (2016): 93–97. https://doi.org/10.1177/1095796016639282.

Szasz, Andrew. *Ecopopulism: Toxic Waste and the Movement for Environmental Justice*. Minneapolis: University of Minnesota Press, 1994.

Sze, Julie. *Noxious New York: The Racial Politics of Urban Health and Environmental Justice*. Cambridge, MA: MIT Press, 2007.

Sze, Julie, Jonathan London, Fraser Shilling, Gerardo Gambirazzio, Trina Filan, and Mary Cadenasso. "Defining and Contesting Environmental Justice: Socio-Natures and the Politics of Scale in the Delta." *Antipode* 41, no. 4 (2009): 807–43. https://doi.org/10.1111/j.1467-8330.2009.00698.x.

Tabuchi, Hiroko. "Biden Administration Cancels Mining Leases near Wilderness Area." *New York Times*, January 26, 2022.

Taggart, Paul A. *Populism*. Buckingham, UK: Open University Press, 2000.

Taylor, Dorceta E. *The Rise of the American Conservation Movement: Power, Privilege, and Environmental Protection*. Durham, NC: Duke University Press, 2016.

———. "Women of Color, Environmental Justice and Ecofeminism." In *Ecofeminism: Women, Culture and Nature*, edited by Karen J. Warren, 38–81. Bloomington: Indiana University Press, 1997.

Teixeira, Ruy, and Joel Rogers. *America's Forgotten Majority: Why the White Working Class Still Matters*. New York: Basic Books, 2000.

Temper, Leah, Federico Demaria, Arnim Scheidel, Daniela Del Bene, and Joan Martinez-Alier. "The Global Environmental Justice Atlas (EJAtlas): Ecological Distribution Conflicts as Forces for Sustainability." *Sustainability Science* 13 (2018): 573–84. https://doi.org/10.1007/s11625-018-0563-4.

Thompson, E. P. *The Making of the English Working Class*. New York: Pantheon Books, 1964.

Threadgold, Steven, David Farrugia, Hedda Askland, Michael Askew, Jo Hanley, Meg Sherval, and Julia Coffey. "Affect, Risk and Local Politics of Knowledge: Changing Land Use in Narrabri, NSW." *Environmental Sociology* 4, no. 4 (2018): 393–404. https://doi.org/10.1080/23251042.2018.1463673.

Tobias, Jimmy. "Meet the Former Koch Adviser Slashing Conservation Safeguards at the Department of the Interior." *Pacific Standard*, January 10, 2018. https://psmag.com.

Tomassoni, David. "Mining Is Us. We Are What We Mine." *Mesabi Daily News*, February 27, 2014.

Treuer, Anton. *Ojibwe in Minnesota*. St Paul: Minnesota Historical Society, 2010.

Tsing, Anna Lowenhaupt. *Friction: An Ethnography of Global Connection*. Princeton, NJ: Princeton University Press, 2005.

———. *The Mushroom at the End of the World: On the Possibility of Life in Capitalist Ruins*. Princeton, NJ: Princeton University Press, 2015.

Turkewitz, Julie. "Bundy Brothers Defend Armed Occupation of Oregon Refuge." *New York Times*, September 29, 2016.

Turner, James Morton. "'The Specter of Environmentalism': Wilderness, Environmental Politics, and the Evolution of the New Right." *Journal of American History* 96, no. 1 (2009): 123–48. https://doi.org/10.2307/27694734.

Twin Metals Minnesota. "About the Project." Accessed April 24, 2018. www.twin-metals.com.

Tyler, Gerald M. "Time for Anti-Mining Accountability." *Mesabi Daily News*, March 1, 2014.

Ulrich-Schad, Jessica D., and Cynthia M. Duncan. "People and Places Left Behind: Work, Culture and Politics in the Rural United States." *Journal of Peasant Studies* 45, no. 1 (2018): 59–79. https://doi.org/10.1080/03066150.2017.1410702.

Ulrich-Schad, Jessica D., and Qin Hua. "Culture Clash? Predictors of Views on Amenity-Led Development and Community Involvement in Rural Recreation Counties." *Rural Sociology* 83, no. 1 (2018): 81–108. https://doi.org/10.1111/ruso.12165.

United Steel Workers Canada. "Steelworkers Step Up Global Campaign against Glencore." September 13, 2007. www.usw.ca.

US Census Bureau. "2011–2015 American Community Survey, 5-Year Estimates." Accessed July 26, 2022. https://data.census.gov.

———. "2013–2017 American Community Survey, 5-Year Estimates." Accessed August 5, 2022. https://data.census.gov.

US Environmental Protection Agency. "About the St. Louis River and Bay AOC." Collections and Lists, March 25, 2015. www.epa.gov.

———. "Hardrock Mining: Environmental Impacts." Office of Water, 2018. www.epa.gov.

———. "National Environmental Policy Act Review Process." Overviews and Factsheets, July 31, 2013. www.epa.gov.

US Geological Survey. *Mineral Commodities Summaries 2016*. Reston, VA: US Department of the Interior, 2016.

———. *Mineral Commodity Summaries 2018*. Washington, DC: US Department of the Interior, January 2018.

———. "Trump Administration Announces Strategy to Strengthen America's Economy, Defense." Press release, US Department of the Interior, June 4, 2019. www.usgs.gov.

US Government Accountability Office. "Environmental Liabilities: Hardrock Mining Cleanup Obligations." Washington, DC: US Government Accountability Office, 2006.

Voyles, Traci Brynne. *Wastelanding: Legacies of Uranium Mining in Navajo Country*. Minneapolis: University of Minnesota Press, 2015.

Wacquant, Loïc. "Making Class: The Middle Class(es) in Social Theory and Social Structure." In *Bringing Class Back In: Contemporary and Historical Perspectives*, edited by Scott G. McNall, Rhonda F. Levine, and Richard Fantasia, 39–63. Boulder, CO: Westview, 1991.

Walgrave, Stefaan, and Joris Verhulst. "Towards 'New Emotional Movements'? A Comparative Exploration into a Specific Movement Type." *Social Movement Studies* 5, no. 3 (2006): 275–304. https://doi.org/10.1080/14742830600991651.

Walker, Peter, and Louise Fortmann. "Whose Landscape? A Political Ecology of the 'Exurban' Sierra." *Cultural Geographies* 10, no. 4 (2003): 469–91. https://doi.org/10.1191/1474474003eu2850a.

Walley, Christine J. "Trump's Election and the 'White Working Class': What We Missed." *American Ethnologist* 44, no. 2 (2017): 231–36. https://doi.org/10.1111/amet.12473.

WaterLegacy. "Oppose the PolyMet NorthMet Sulfide Mine: Protect Environmental Justice, Human Health and Climate Resilience." St. Paul, MN, 2017. https://waterlegacy.org.

Waters, Mary C. *Ethnic Options: Choosing Identities in America*. Berkeley: University of California Press, 1990.

Watt, Laura Alice. *The Paradox of Preservation: Wilderness and Working Landscapes at Point Reyes National Seashore*. Berkeley: University of California Press, 2016.

Weszkalnys, Gisa. "A Doubtful Hope: Resource Affect in a Future Oil Economy." *Journal of the Royal Anthropological Institute* 22, no. 51 (2016): 127–46. https://doi.org/10.1111/1467-9655.12397.

Wheeler, Rebecca. "Local History as Productive Nostalgia? Change, Continuity and Sense of Place in Rural England." *Social & Cultural Geography* 18, no. 4 (2017): 466–86. https://doi.org/10.1080/14649365.2016.1189591.

———. "Mining Memories in a Rural Community: Landscape, Temporality and Place Identity." *Journal of Rural Studies* 36 (2014): 22–32. https://doi.org/10.1016/j.jrurstud.2014.06.005.

Whieldon, Esther, and Annie Snider. "Trump's Interior Pick Lifts Outdoors Groups." *Politico*, December 15, 2016. www.politico.com.

White, Erik. *2017 Regional Profile: Economic Development Region 3—Northeast Minnesota*. Duluth: Minnesota Department of Employment and Economic Development, August 1, 2017.

White, Jonathan. "Climate Change and the Generational Timescape." *Sociological Review* 65, no. 4 (2017): 763–78. https://doi.org/10.1111/1467-954X.12397.

White, Richard. "'Are You an Environmentalist or Do You Work for a Living?': Work and Nature." In *Uncommon Ground: Rethinking the Human Place in Nature*, edited by William Cronon, 171–85. New York: Norton, 1995.

Whyte, Kyle Powys. "Settler Colonialism, Ecology, and Environmental Injustice." *Environment and Society* 9, no. 1 (2018): 125–44. https://doi.org/10.3167/ares.2018.090109.

Widick, Richard. *Trouble in the Forest: California's Redwood Timber Wars*. Minneapolis: University of Minnesota Press, 2009.

Wilder Research. "Location Profiles: Ely Data." Minnesota Compass. Accessed July 24, 2022. www.mncompass.org.

———. "Location Profiles: Iron Range Resources and Rehabilitation Service Area Data." Minnesota Compass. Accessed July 24, 2022. www.mncompass.org.

———. "Minnesota's Population: All Minnesotans." Minnesota Compass. Accessed July 24, 2022. www.mncompass.org.

Woods, Michael, Jon Anderson, Steven Guilbert, and Suzie Watkin. "'The Country(side) Is Angry': Emotion and Explanation in Protest Mobilization." *Social & Cultural Geography* 13, no. 6 (2012): 567–85. https://doi.org/10.1080/14649365.2012.704643.

World Health Organization. "Mercury and Health." 2018. www.who.int.

Wuthnow, Robert. *The Left Behind: Decline and Rage in Small-Town America*. Princeton, NJ: Princeton University Press, 2018. https://doi.org/10.2307/j.ctvc773q2.

Zavestoski, Stephen, Frank Mignano, Kate Agnello, Francine Darroch, and Katy Abrams. "Toxicity and Complicity: Explaining Consensual Community Response to a Chronic Technological Disaster." *Sociological Quarterly* 43, no. 3 (2002): 385–406. https://doi.org/10.1111/j.1533-8525.2002.tb00054.x.

Zerubavel, Eviatar. *Time Maps: Collective Memory and the Social Shape of the Past*. Chicago: University of Chicago Press, 2004.

INDEX

Page numbers in *italics* indicate Tables and Photos

ABOUT THE AUTHOR

ERIK KOJOLA is Assistant Professor of Sociology in the Department of Sociology and Anthropology at Texas Christian University. He is the author of numerous articles and book chapters on environmental politics, labor, political ecology, and extractive industries.